STEAMED GREENS FOR THE SPIRIT

Your Journey Into Total Wellness...

With the Three Pillars of Health,
Seven Transformational Questions,
And 46 Action Steps to Consider Now

©2004 John M. Kalb, M.S., D.C.

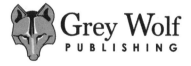

Grey Wolf
PUBLISHING

Ashland, Oregon

Grey Wolf Publishing

450 Siskiyou Blvd.
Ashland, OR 97520

Phone: 541-488-3001

This book is designed to assist you in finding greater health and wellness in your life. It is not meant to diagnose, treat or replace any necessary medical care. Each person and situation is unique. If you are under the care of a health professional, then check with them before starting any activity mentioned in this book that could impact your condition.

All the names of patients and clients used in this book are fictitious but the stories are true.

First North American Edition (Soft cover)
Printed in Canada on 100% Post Consumer Recycled Paper

Book cover design by Gaelyn Larrick
Back cover photo by Pam Danielle Photography

ISBN: 0-9749235-1-6

Dedication

This book is dedicated to the loving memory of my father.
He inspired me in many ways,
including becoming a doctor and healer,
in part because of his many lifetime health problems.
On his deathbed he told me that I had saved his life with nutrition
and given him ten more good years.

This book is also dedicated to health seekers everywhere.

Contents

List of Baby Steps	vii
Acknowledgments	ix
Introduction	xi

PART I: THE WELLNESS PROCESS:
SEVEN QUESTIONS TO TRANSFORM YOUR HEALTH

Chapter 1: More Health Now	1
Chapter 2: Impact	3
Chapter 3: The Health You Want	5
Chapter 4: Baby Steps to Health	7
Chapter 5: Excuses, Excuses…	9
Chapter 6: The Hidden Risk	11
Chapter 7: Just Do It!	19
The Wellness Process™ Worksheet	21

PART II: THE THREE PILLARS OF WELLNESS

Chapter 8: A Simple Model Of Wellness-The Three Pillars	27
Chapter 9: The Structural Pillar	31
Chapter 10: The Pillar Of Biochemistry	45
Chapter 11: The Pillar Of The Mind	75
EPILOGUE: A Sustainable Future:	
Healthy People=Healthy Planet	105

PART III: APPENDICES

A. Recommended Books and Websites	109
B. Other Resources	115
C. Endnotes	125
D. Dr Kalb's Bio and Philosophy	127

LIST OF BABY STEPS

#1 Exercising Optimally 32

#2 Stretching Program 32

#3 Strength and Power Building 32

#4 Exercising Balance 33

#5 Sculpting Posture 34

#6 Sleep Time and Power Napping 35

#7 Deep Three-Part Breathing 36

#8 Experiencing Massage 37

#9 The Training Cycle 38

#10 Prolonging Pleasure 39

#11 Performing Kegel Contractions 39

#12 Contrast Showering 40

#13 Finding a Chiropractor 42

#14 Solving Chronic Pain 44

#15 Drinking Lots of Water 48

#16 Kicking the Coffee Habit 49

#17 Eating Natural and Organic 50

#18 Minimizing the Use of White Sugar 50

#19 Balancing Proteins, Carbohydrates and Fat 51

#20 Eating "Good" Fats 52

#21 Eating Lots of Veggies 53

#22 Supplementing For Health 55

#23 Eating Raw Food and Enzymes 57

#24 Enhancing Digestion 60

#25 Allergy-Free Cleansing 65

#26 Passing Safely Through Menopause 67

#27 Facing the Challenge of Andropause 68

#28 Experimenting Safely with Natural Hormones 70

#29 Reviewing Your Meds 73

#30 Creating Affirmation 77

#31 Reframing 79

#32 Forgiving 81

#33 Mindfully Meditating 82

#34 Practicing Relaxation 83

LIST OF BABY STEPS (Continued)

#35 Sharing Three Positives Before a Negative   **85**

#36 Releasing Withholds   **86**

#37 Being Accountable   **87**

#38 Committing   **87**

#39 Victim/Victor Reframing   **90**

#40 Reclaiming Your Power   **92**

#41 Confronting Boredom   **92**

#42 Identifying What Matters Most – Core Values   **95**

#43 Setting Honest Boundaries   **96**

#44 Emotional Stretching   **97**

#45 Refocusing Technique   **100**

#46 Embracing Death as Ally   **103**

Acknowledgments

I have many people to thank for helping me complete this book. First and foremost I want to express my deepest gratitude to my beautiful wife Shari, who has helped me in many ways, not the least of which was transcribing and laying out the book. I want to thank the men in my men's group for nurturing and supporting the very idea of this book from the beginning, especially Len Snyder and Tej Steiner. I also want to thank Bill Kauth and the Mankind Project for making my men's group possible. I am very grateful for the two women coaches in my life, Elizabeth Austin and Denise Byron. I am incredibly indebted to my writing coach, Craig Comstock and my two editors, Anni Powell and Dee Birkes. I want to thank my close friend and book cover designer Gaelyn Larrick, for mentoring me in many ways and also my buddy, Will Wilkinson, for moral support, layout and publishing information. In addition I want to acknowledge Dan Sheehan for all his support and for the finishing touches on the book cover. I also appreciate my office manager Penelope Dews for keeping my office running smoothly, giving me the confidence to devote much time to this project. I want to acknowledge two long time friends Allan Weisbard and Paul O'Brien for seeing the best in me and for their honest feedback.

INTRODUCTION

Assumptions

This book is based on the following assumptions:
- Most people want to be healthy.
- Most people are aware that lifestyle habits are a major factor in creating, maintaining or destroying health.
- Most people already know of healthy lifestyle habits they want to start doing.
- Most people are not doing them.

This disconnection is why I wrote this book. **If you are like most people, you don't need more information about what to do, you just need help getting started doing it.** I have developed a way you can move beyond your resistance and do what it takes to create greater health in your life.

The Beauty of It

The beauty of this process is that it is simple, effective and gets you moving. I have found that just getting started is the key. You can become energized and ride an upward spiral of positive feedback, which makes you feel better about yourself and reinforces continuing the process. More energy is then generated as health benefits begin manifesting.

Simple things like walking regularly, drinking more water, breathing more deeply, meditating or eating more fruits and vegetables can make a huge difference in your health and vitality.

Many people find that if they can keep up an activity for about three weeks, then it becomes almost effortless as a well-ingrained, positive habit. Then if desired, the process can be repeated to include additional health habits.

The Real Problem

If this is so easy, then why doesn't everyone just do it and get healthier? Well, the scary thing is, by most standards we as a society are getting sicker and sicker, even as we live longer and longer. Western medicine is good at diagnosing and treating disease but not at prevention and wellness.

So what's the real problem? Is it that we are lazy, ignorant and don't have the motivation? **NO!** It's my contention that we have "mental blocks" or hidden limiting beliefs that keep us from getting on the upward spiral to health. Beyond all the excuses and rationalizations, once these obstacles are uncovered, they lose their power over us. We can then make new choices and get moving in a healthy direction. This is crucial: **for a wellness program to be successful it can't demand too much time, effort or discipline.**

More Good News

More good news: this process is not about changing yourself. That can be really hard to do and raises significant inner resistance. The ego will dig in for all it's worth when it feels threatened and change sounds threatening to the ego. Instead, *you can easily just get started by taking simple action steps that will build to a health-promoting life.* This is done by setting a new positive intention to become healthier, selecting an easily obtainable goal and then using your natural curiosity to uncover and neutralize limiting beliefs or mental blocks. Once you take your first "baby step" you get that sweet taste of success. The process then becomes self-perpetuating and wellness is yours.

A Limiting Belief

I have a patient whom I will call Peter who could not seem to keep his weight in check or keep from slouching more and more each year. (All the names used in this book are fictitious, but the stories are true). Peter's father died at the age of 53. As Peter approached this age part of him felt, "Why bother to be healthy since I am going to die at age 53 anyway?" After doing the Wellness Process™ and uncovering this limiting belief, Peter was able to make new choices about overcoming his genetic weaknesses instead of giving in to them. He now feels he deserves to surpass his father's life span and his father would have wanted it that way as well. Peter has finally been able to lose weight and his posture has improved reflecting an increased sense of self-worth.

How to Get the Most Out of this Book

1. Feel free to implement new health activities or baby steps into your lifestyle, including those from Part II, The Three Pillars of Wellness that produce little or no resistance.

2. Use Part I, The Wellness Process™: Seven Questions to Transform Your Health, to implement the one baby step that seems the most important or helpful to you that **does** generate resistance. However, make sure it is still easily attainable so that you benefit from an early success.

3. Use Part I to implement other baby steps as needed once you have turned the previous baby step into a positive health habit.

4. You can also use Part II and Part III (Appendices) as reference and inspiration for choosing additional health activities in the future.

5. **Before you start Part I, I recommend that you have a pen or pencil in hand and at least 45 minutes of undisturbed time. (It can also be done in several shorter sessions).**

When you are ready to find out how this process works for you, turn to the next chapter and let's get started!

PART I

THE WELLNESS PROCESS™:

SEVEN QUESTIONS TO TRANSFORM YOUR HEALTH

CHAPTER I
MORE HEALTH NOW

The first wealth is health.
Emerson

Just about everyone with whom I have ever talked has some health issues and desires to be healthier. This is understandable as over 64% of the U.S. population is overweight,[1] and the U.S. lags behind other industrialized nations in health ratings. Out of the 13 most developed nations, the U.S. ranks last in infant mortality and third from the bottom in age-adjusted mortality (life expectancy).[2] In a recent study by the World Health Organization, the U.S. ranked 15th out of 25 other industrialized nations in overall health.[3] We also spend much more money on health care per year ($3,925 per person) than any other country,[4] even as our system is failing us. Increasing numbers of people are seeking out natural and alternative methods of health care. Many Americans have become dissatisfied and disillusioned with standard medical care and are searching for a better approach. So right now answer this question:
Are you as healthy as you want to be?
☐ No (Thanks for the honesty! Proceed.)
☐ Yes (Congratulations! You may not need to proceed.)

If you are like most people, then you answered "No," you are not as healthy as you want to be. That's fine, because I am confident that if you follow through with this process, your health will improve significantly.
What are the definitions of health and wellness anyway? Health is defined in <u>Dorland's Medical Dictionary</u> as, "…optimal physical, mental and social well being and not merely the absence of disease or infirmity." <u>Merriam-Webster</u> (on-line) has it as being, "…sound in body, mind and spirit." Note that health not only spans the body/mind spectrum but also encompasses the social and spiritual as well! The <u>Merriam-Webster</u> (on-line) definition of wellness is, "…being in good health *especially as an actively sought goal.*" (emphasis added.) I define wellness as simply the pathway or journey into health. This is very freeing and does not exclude us from wellness because of our

current physical condition or our genetics. **Wellness is a process, not a destination.** Even a disease-ridden couch potato can make a decision; set a new intention and start moving in the direction of increased health, thus meeting my definition of wellness.

The above definition of health, as optimal physical, mental and social well being, may in fact be unattainable. It's crucial to redefine health for ourselves. Let's call it **excellent health**.

Throughout the first part of this book I strongly recommend that you take your time and jot down your answers to the questions in the spaces provided. Please don't rush ahead just reading the questions. The value comes in actually answering them. The effort you put forth now will pay you back many dividends later!

What would excellent health be like for you?

_____

_____

_____

_____

_____.

The next step in this process is to look at the costs or negative impacts of your lack of excellent health. Read on.

CHAPTER II
IMPACT

Health is so necessary to all of the duties,
as well as the pleasures of life,
that the crime of squandering it is equal to the folly.
Samuel Johnson

Since help is on the way, I am going to ask you to be willing to look at the costs or negative impacts of not being as healthy as you want to be. It's common for people, especially optimists, to want to paint a rosy picture about their health. That will not be helpful here. On the other hand, you pessimists or "whiners" will have no problem with the following questions. So let your positive filters down and take a good, hard look at your current health status and in all honesty answer the following question.

What are the costs of your lack of excellent health on your life?

_____

_____

_____

_____

_____.

Look at your health from a slightly different perspective and answer this question.

What can't you do?

_____

_____

_____

_____

_____.

Finally, I want to help to you get in touch with what's really important about this for you.

At its worst, which of your core values does your lack of excellent health threaten?

_____

_____

_____

_____

_____.

When you are satisfied with your answers to these questions and/or have spent a reasonable amount of time on them, then move on to Chapter III and we will look at the benefits of getting the health you want!

CHAPTER III
THE HEALTH YOU WANT

In this chapter I want to help you generate some excitement about the benefits of becoming truly healthy. While working on this chapter it is helpful if you free up your imagination and don't worry about being practical or realistic. The next chapter will be the time and place for that. Now, I invite you to have some fun with this and let go of any constraints or inhibitions you may be feeling.

If you currently have an illness or disease of a chronic or genetic nature, it may not be realistic to imagine being completely cured; but I am going to ask you to do that anyway! Remember, wellness is a journey, not a destination. So anything you can do to gain inspiration and take action in a positive direction increases wellness. If you have an "incurable disease," living well in the present and increasing your mental, emotional and spiritual health is not only possible but extraordinarily important. Even on your deathbed, by facing the end of this life with grace and dignity, you can embrace wellness.

What would be the benefits of actually achieving the health you want?

_____

_____

_____

_____

_____.

Now sit back, relax, and enjoy this next part. During the guided visualization that follows, give yourself the opportunity to pause and follow each instruction thoroughly. Take a few slow deep breaths, make sure you are comfortable and let yourself relax.

Imagine, at some future time - say a year or two from now - that you have achieved the health and vitality you want. Let your imagination run free and actually see and feel what it would be like. You also may be able to remember a time when you did feel really good, healthy and full of calm energy. Notice the expression on your face and your body posture. What sounds are you hearing and what do you imagine other people are saying to you? What positive things are you saying to yourself? What are you doing? Now feel free to add any fantasy touches to make it just the way you want it to be. Imagine yourself doing something or succeeding in a way that you have always wanted to but haven't been able to, because of lack of health or energy. Take your time with this. Take another few deep, relaxing breaths and enjoy this image and the state you are in right now. When you are ready… slowly come back to the present and from this space answer the next two questions.

What would you be able to do or achieve that you haven't yet been able to?

_____

_____

_____

_____

_____.

At a deeper level, which of your core values would excellent health enhance?

_____

_____

_____

_____

_____.

CHAPTER IV
BABY STEPS TO HEALTH

A journey of a thousand miles begins with the first step.

Lao Tzu

Here is an important question for you at this point in the process: **Is there a health activity or habit that you would like to start or follow through with but haven't yet?**

□ **Yes (Great, proceed!)**
□ **No (Please go back to question #1 and start over, or read Part II of this book).**

I recommend that you pick something that is eminently attainable so you make succeeding at it easy. The energy you get from having a small success will help keep you going until it becomes a habit. I have found this principle to be very helpful.

Here is an example of how hidden resistance can create self-sabotage and lead to setting too high of a goal. Natalie had a few pounds to lose and was bothered by some minor knee pain. Knowing that swimming is a good exercise for the knee, Natalie decided to join the YMCA and start swimming on a regular basis. Each time she returned for an appointment, she had a different excuse about why she hadn't started swimming. Upon questioning, it turned out that her mother had been a competitive swimmer. Natalie had never enjoyed it as a child and she felt guilty about that. She had a limiting belief about swimming that she could never do it good enough to get her mother's approval, so why bother? Natalie had sabotaged herself by choosing a giant step rather than a baby one, thus setting herself up for failure. After doing The Wellness Process™ she chose to do some simple knee exercises and ride a stationary bike. After about three months she had lost over ten pounds and her knee was improved, not only from the exercise but also from having less weight to support. Setting unreasonably high goals is a common form of self-sabotage, which I affectionately call "biting off more than you can chew."

Overcoming Inertia

Typically, when I have a patient with chronic low back pain, I recommend a home exercise program tailored to their specific needs. If on their subsequent visit I find that they haven't started yet, then I recommend just one or two exercises at a time to help overcome their inertia. I then make the suggestion that we go through this process.

With that introduction, I invite you now to pick a simple activity or behavior that you have wanted to do but haven't started yet or have not followed through with consistently. Again, I want to remind you to pick something that is a baby step for you and not a huge project. Remember the saying of Lao Tzu quoted at the beginning of this chapter. Make your goal something you can achieve easily and plunge right in.

Next, I would like you to be specific with your action step. For instance, "I walk three or four times per week for at least 30 minutes," or "I eat better so I only have desert once or twice a week, and I eat a fresh salad and a piece of fruit daily." Other examples might be: "I take some quiet time every day and remember to breathe deeply and relax my shoulders," or "I am joining that yoga class and go three times a week." What I am encouraging you to do is move from a large, vague goal of being healthier, to a single specific action step you can start immediately. It's O.K. to brainstorm several ideas, then chose one. A well stated baby step is clear, simple and measurable and is an empowering call to action.

How can you state this as a baby step in an easily attainable and specific manner?

_____

_____

_____

_____

_____.

Again, I strongly advise you to actually write down your responses to the questions! All we have to do now is move past any excuses by uncovering your hidden resistance. Please proceed.

8

CHAPTER V
EXCUSES, EXCUSES . . .

Now I would like you to look at the reasons or rationalizations you have used in the past for not starting or following through with your health activity or habit. I hope to show you next that these are not the real reasons, so don't be attached to them or to any shame or embarrassment you might be feeling. This is perfectly normal. I know most of us have made lots of excuses in the past for not getting things done. I, for one, admit to having been a master procrastinator, coming from a long line of procrastinators. My father was an English professor and a writer, but he only published a few works because he could not overcome his "writer's block." I have come up with all kinds of excuses for not finishing this book, and I notice that they are similar to the excuses I use for not exercising as often as I'd like. "I'm too tired." " I'm not inspired." "I'm not good enough." "I don't deserve it." " I'll do it later when I feel better." " I don't have enough time, other things are more important right now." After doing this process with myself, one of the things I realized was that out of "love" for my deceased father, I did not want to surpass him and be more successful or more productive. Realizing that my love for him will not be diminished if I am more successful than he was has helped me write this book. It is obvious that I have been able to finish writing this book and I still have just as much love for my dad. *I know from personal experience that this process works.*

As a prelude to letting go, neutralizing and moving past your excuses, I would like you to answer the following question: **What's stopping you? Please list all your reasons or excuses here:**

_____

_____

_____

_____

_____.

CHAPTER VI
THE HIDDEN RISK

A Perfect Example

Here is a perfect example of identifying a hidden risk from doing this process with an acquaintance of mine named Sally. She is an attractive young woman who is moderately overweight and very concerned about her poor body image. She also has other health issues associated with her excess weight and her eating habits. She saw the potential benefits of losing weight and becoming healthier but she was a confirmed chocoholic and sugar addict. She tried and failed many times to give them up. Finally she got in touch with the real hidden risk for her of actually losing the weight. She was afraid that she would attract too much male attention and become promiscuous. The dialogue went like this:

"So Sally, what would be the risk of eating better and losing weight?"

"Well, if I actually lost the weight, I might become too attractive."

"Okay, so what's the risk for you of becoming too attractive?"

"Then men would keep bothering me."

"What's the risk of that?"

"I am afraid that I would become distracted from my goals."

"What's the risk of that?"

"Oh my gosh, I'm afraid I would enjoy it, lose control, and start sleeping around."

"So, what's the risk of that?"

"I would lose all self worth and feel like dying."

At this point she dropped her eyes and started rocking back and forth slightly, thus exhibiting a *truth response*. **A truth response is an external and observable manifestation of having an "Aha" experience or feeling a flash of insight.** It usually involves a subtle reaction such as exhaling deeply (sighing), closing the eyes, rocking back and forth slightly or even exhibiting a startle reaction and momentarily freezing up and looking like a "deer caught in the headlights."

She felt safer with the extra weight "protecting her from men." Once this mental block was out in the open for her to see and evaluate, it lost some of its power over her. She was now willing to face the unlikely risk of possibly becoming promiscuous. She began to replace the chocolate and sugar with fruit and to eat more protein to balance her blood sugar. During the Wellness Process™ she got to the deep place of being able to experience *the horns of the dilemma*. **This is a situation or predicament where two diametrically opposed choices are both fraught with risks,** often but not always the same risk. When I asked her what was the risk of becoming promiscuous, she said she would lose all self-esteem and die emotionally. The bottom line risk is often found to be facing our core fears of lack of self worth (death) or abandonment (disconnection). She was simultaneously aware that the risk of **not** eating properly and losing the weight was shortened life, in effect, death as well. So on each horn of the dilemma, she had to face death. "If I don't eat right, I might die early, and if I do eat right, I might die emotionally." She courageously chose to eat right and face her irrational fear that she might die. As you might expect, not only did she live, but she was also able to achieve the benefits of eating better and losing weight.

Another way to look at this case is through the understanding of *secondary gain*. In other words, what did Sally get out of keeping the weight on? How did it serve her? She was using the weight as a shield or buffer to protect her from men, sort of like a booby prize. Secondary gain is like that, it may not sound like such a great deal, but *it does serve a psychological need.*

To help uncover any secondary gain or self-destructive behaviors you may have, answer these questions.

What do you get out of your lack of excellent health? How does that work for you? What is your payoff or secondary gain?

_____

_____

_____

_____

_____.

<u>**Self-destructive behavior or self-sabotage is what we do to maintain our secondary gain.**</u> Sally had tried and failed at many diets for this reason. Despite her best intentions, she could never follow through and always let something get in the way. The **risk** for her was to give up her secondary gain, her protective shield of excess weight, and to face her irrational fear of promiscuity, etc.

Our Emotional Predicament

Where does hidden resistance come from anyway? Every one of us is unique, and still we face a common psychological dilemma. One theory explaining this says that we all come into this world with the same basic biological and psychological needs (see <u>A General</u> <u>Theory of Love</u> by Thomas Lewis, M.D., Fari Amini, M.D. and Richard Lannon, M.D.). As infants and then toddlers, we absolutely require nurturing and love to thrive, even to develop properly. Unfortunately, few, if any of us, receive this love unconditionally all the time from our parents or primary care givers. This lack of love produces pain or hurt on a deep emotional level and occurs before we learn to talk. We may then react to this pain with fear and this pain/fear cycle is repeated many times. Eventually anger and sadness develop and their expression can be unacceptable to our caregivers. Control and depression then develop as defense mechanisms, and finally, when we are old enough, we blame ourselves for this whole dynamic and feel shame. **At our core we take on the wound of feeling unworthy, abandoned or a combination of both.**

During this painful process, *the young innocent one will try to avoid the pain by developing an ego strategy to win love and approval from the parents.* This is the birth of what is called negative love and it takes the form of one of four dynamics: (1) copying key behaviors of our parents; (2) copying the way another important person treats one of our parents; or when older rebelling and (3) actually doing the opposite of (1); or (4) doing the opposite of (2). (See Kani Comstock's book <u>Journey Into Love</u>.) This whole constellation of emotions and behavioral strategies is a major contributor to our ego identity. The good news is that it allows us to survive childhood and grow up to be a more or less successful adult. The bad news is that we become inauthentic as we cover up our core pain and fear of being unworthy and/or of being abandoned.

This is our emotional predicament as humans. One way to heal this is to allow ourselves to become aware of it and to learn how to love and forgive <u>ourselves</u> at ever-deepening levels.

The Horns of the Dilemma

So what keeps us stuck and blocks us from creating the health we truly want? Are we lazy, ignorant or stupid? **<u>No!</u>** It is hidden resistance that often involves protecting and maintaining our secondary gain, as was demonstrated in the previous example of Sally. It can also involve avoiding looking at our deepest fears. **Our core fears of unworthiness and abandonment are often manifested in present time as fear of success and/or fear of failure.** For most of the people who have done the Wellness Process™, these hidden risks were often learned from our parents as patterns of negative love. Once they are laid bare, some of their power is discharged. We are then able to break free and achieve greater levels of health and well being by taking one baby step at a time. In some of my most successful cases, my client or patient has gotten to the place of clearly seeing the horns of the dilemma and then was able to move forward almost effortlessly. Read on for an excellent example of this.

Steamed Greens For The Spirit

Gloria is a very self-aware person who has done much inner work. I suspected that she would get a lot out of this process even though she lived a reasonably healthy lifestyle. She did state that she wanted greater levels of health and energy for herself and she also wanted to improve her diet by eating less sugar. I suggested, and she agreed, to eat a cup of steamed greens at least six days a week. I have found this, along with adequate protein, to be an almost universal antidote for sugar craving. When I asked her what her risk was, she was vaguely aware of discomfort around having the increased energy that improved health would bring.

"So what would be the risk of having more energy?" I innocently asked. Light bulbs started popping for her. She realized she had a fear of success that this additional healthy energy might bring out. Then I asked her, "What is the risk for you of being more successful?"

"Ah," I heard the deep sigh of her truth response. "I am afraid people won't like me and I'll be rejected and left alone." We had struck pay dirt! *She had identified her core fear of abandonment.*

I then asked her to put out one hand and in it place (1), her desire to be healthier and have more energy by eating steamed greens regularly and (2), the associated core level fear of being abandoned. Next I asked her to put out her other hand and I asked, "What's the emotional risk for you if you don't achieve the health and energy you want?"

She almost exploded as she said, "I'm afraid I'll get sick and be abandoned anyway." Eureka! Both horns of the dilemma were identical and represented her deepest fear.

I then had her weigh her two hands and appreciate her predicament.

"So it looks like the same big risk either way; get healthier and risk your fear of success and abandonment, or, on the other hand, get sick and face abandonment. Are you willing to take the risk and follow through with your new health habit? It looks like either way you have to face the same risk."

"It's a no-brainer." she exclaimed, "I have the same risk on either side. I would rather go for the health and risk being more successful."

What was the baby step she had chosen, her action step? Who would have thought that committing to eating steamed greens could lead to such a deep and profound emotional awakening? This is a truly classic case of *seizing the horns of the dilemma.* Gloria has followed through with more coaching sessions and continues to eat her greens. She also became aware that her fear of success was a negative love pattern learned from her father, who was a genuine genius but failed miserably in most areas of his life. Out of love for her dad, Gloria adopted a fear of success. This process was the beginning of a profound transformation for Gloria and her spirit was truly energized. Who knows? *Steamed greens for the spirit?* It just might be true.

Another Example

Sylvia had chosen a simple action step of taking 15 minutes for herself each day to do relaxation and breathing exercises. She put off doing this for some time and it was obvious to me that there was a lot of hidden resistance. When I asked her what the risk was she said, "What risk? There is none."

I replied, "Since you have been wanting to do this for some time but haven't yet, there must be a risk." To help her get in touch with the risk I asked her to state her main excuses.

She said, "I am just too busy, I don't have the time, I wouldn't be able to get as much stuff done."

"I see." I said, "So what would happen if you didn't get so much done."

After a long pause she finally said, "I might get in trouble, and people wouldn't like me."

I then asked her, "What would be the risk of that?" At this point she looked startled and confused, her eyes dropped, and she whispered something about "being rejected." I knew we were on the money because of her truth response.

"So," I said, "your hidden risk of taking 15 minutes for yourself is that you might be rejected by other people."

"That sounds crazy," she said. "Actually I would probably do a better job and get more done because I would be more relaxed and less stressed."

"That's probably true," I said, "but that irrational fear has real power over you. On the other hand, what would be the risk if you don't change, not taking a little time for yourself, and continuing to be stressed?"

"Well, I might start making more mistakes and get rejected anyway." she said.

"Exactly!" I said, "There are risks either way. Stay the same and risk being rejected, or take time for yourself and also risk being rejected. It looks like a no-brainer for you to risk taking time for yourself and seeing what happens." As in the previous case, both horns of the dilemma were the same.

In the case of Sylvia the secondary gain was not that clear to her. What does she get out of being stressed and not taking time for herself? Perhaps her self-esteem is wrapped up in how much she gets done, like a workaholic. Also, there could be a bit of a martyr complex going on, as it is popularly called. I am sure most of you know or have known someone who is always doing for other people, never for themselves. They often feed off other's guilt and their own self-pity. To become healthier it's valuable for these folks to be willing to look at giving up some of their secondary gain and taking time for themselves. It is often helpful for them to consider that they are a person, too, and giving to themselves can be just as valid as giving to others.

If you haven't hit your own truth response or had an "Aha" experience, relax. Don't worry. You can still move ahead with your chosen baby step and generate increased health and wellness. For some people just looking at their issues is enough to break up the logjam and motivate them into action. You can keep these questions in mind over the next several weeks as you move forward with your health activity and more understanding may come. If not, at least you will be moving.

Now ask yourself: **What is the risk of actually obtaining the health you want? In other words, what might you have to face, give up or change?**

_____

_____

_____

_____

_____.

As you have seen from the examples above: **Go deeper and keep asking yourself, "What would be the risk of that?" until you hit the bottom line and feel a "truth response."**

_____

_____

_____

_____

_____.

At this point it may be helpful for you to demonstrate this physically. So put out one hand and in it "put" or visualize the health you want and the baby step you have chosen. When you have done that, then put your bottom line risk of obtaining it there as well. This could be fear of success or failure, too much responsibility, burn-out, lack of self worth, fear of abandonment or death, etc.

Now hold out your other hand and put the answer to this question there: **What would be the emotional risk for you of <u>not</u> achieving the health you want?**

_____

_____

_____

_____

_____.

Now, weigh your two hands and feel your predicament!

CHAPTER VII
JUST DO IT!

This is the final step! I would like you to honestly face the predicament in which you may now find yourself. If you don't do something different, then you run the risk of experiencing your health decline, perhaps dying sooner and missing out on the joys and benefits of greater health. If you are willing to begin to establish a new health habit, then you face the hidden risk you may have uncovered in the last chapter. So what are you going to do? Either way there are risks. Now the hidden risk you uncovered may be irrational and not come to pass; but as long as you don't face and acknowledge it, the power it has over you stays real.

This reminds me of body surfing in the ocean at the shore break. When a big wave comes in, doing nothing can be disastrous. You must either dive with it and ride it in towards the shore, or turn and face it and dive under the wave as it passes over you. **Turn now and face the wave, the horns of your dilemma.** Stay stuck in the old patterns, or face the fears of embracing the new. Stay stuck and die, or face the unknown and possibly die. Remember the inspiring words of Patrick Henry, "Give me liberty or give me death."

You may also be feeling just the opposite of that right now as well! If you choose to stay where you are, then you should actually honor yourself for needing to be safe and to move slowly. If you **are** ready to begin something new, then I strongly recommend that you take action in that direction immediately. There is tremendous power in making a decision and acting on it right away.

The Power of Commitment
. . . the moment one definitely commits oneself,
Providence moves too.
All sorts of things occur to help
that would never otherwise have occurred.
A whole stream of events issues from the decision
raising in one's favor all manner of unforeseen incidents,
meetings and material assistance,
which no one would have dreamed possible.

W.H. Murray

Are you ready to face the risk, irrational though it may be, and move ahead with your activity? Check all that apply.

☐ **YES, I understand my emotional risks and/or I am willing to face them.**

☐ **NO, I don't understand, I need more time, or I don't choose to face them right now.**

☐ **YES, I choose to proceed with my health activity, take a baby step and just do it!**

In the famous words of the Nike slogan, "Just do it." If you have not chosen to move ahead, then I invite you to redo this part of the book from the beginning at some later time and see what happens. You have nothing to lose. For the rest of you, go ahead and get started and congratulations! During the next three weeks, while you are establishing the new habit and beginning to feel the benefits, I recommend that you read PART II - THE THREE PILLARS OF WELLNESS, and consider picking another health practice from one of the other two pillars (the three being **structural, biochemical and mental**). Once your new habit is established, if you have resistance or hesitate taking your next baby step, then redoing the Wellness Process™ will help you take that next step. This cycle can be repeated until your lifestyle truly supports your values and health goals.

Immediately following is a worksheet containing all seven questions for your use. I recommend photocopying it with my permission for repeated use in the future. I see this as a lifetime voyage of discovery, this journey into wellness - getting healthy, staying healthy and aging gracefully. Good luck and *may the blessings of health be with you!*

THE WELLNESS PROCESS™ WORKSHEET

1a. Are you as healthy as you want to be?
   ☐ **NO** (Thanks for the honesty, proceed.)
   ☐ **YES** (Congratulations, you may not need to proceed.)

1b. What would excellent health be like for you?

_____

_____

_____

_____.

2a. What are the costs of your lack of excellent health on your life?

_____

_____

_____

_____.

2b. What can't you do?

_____

_____

_____

_____.

2c. At its worst, which of your core values does your lack of excellent health threaten?

_____

_____

_____

_____.

3a. What would be the benefits of actually achieving the health you want?

_____

_____

_____

_____.

3b. What would you be able to do or achieve that you haven't yet been able to do?

_____

_____

_____

_____.

3c. At a deeper level, which of your core values would excellent health enhance?

_____

_____

_____

_____.

4a. Is there a health activity or habit you would like to start or follow with but haven't yet?
     ☐ **YES** (Great proceed!)
     ☐ **NO** (Please go back to question #1, start over or read PART II of this book.)

4b. Can you state this as a baby step, in an easily attainable and
     specific manner?

_____

_____

_____

_____.

5. What is stopping you? Please list all your reasons or excuses here.

_____

_____

_____

_____.

6a. What do you get out of your lack of excellent health? How does
     that work for you? What is your payoff or secondary gain?

_____

_____

_____

_____.

6b. What is the risk of actually obtaining the health you want? In
     other words, what might you have to face, give up or change?

_____

_____

_____

_____.

6c. Go deeper and keep asking yourself, "What would be the risk of that?" until you hit the bottom line and feel a *truth response*.

_____

_____

_____

_____.

6d. On the other hand, what would be the emotional risk for you of **not** achieving the health you want?

_____

_____

_____

_____.

7. Are you ready to face the risk, irrational though it may be, and move ahead with your activity? Check all that apply.
    ☐ **YES**, I understand my emotional risks and/or I am willing to face them.
    ☐ **NO**, I don't understand, I need more time or I don't choose to face them right now.
    ☐ **YES**, I choose to move ahead with my health activity, take a baby step and just do it!

PART II

THE THREE PILLARS OF WELLNESS

CHAPTER VIII
A SIMPLE MODEL OF WELLNESS –
THE THREE PILLARS

The doctor of the future will give no medicine,
but will interest his patients in the care of the human frame,
in diet and in the cause and prevention of disease.
Thomas Edison

The three pillars of wellness are **structural, biochemical and mental**. This is a useful simplification of an obvious complexity. The structural pillar includes those areas of life dealing with our bodies in a more or less mechanical fashion, such as exercise, posture, breathing and physical medicine. The biochemical pillar includes diet, nutrition, supplements, digestion, medication and those things directly affecting our body chemistry. The mental pillar includes the psychological, the emotional and the spiritual. All three pillars or domains are interdependent and affect our overall health and well being. For example, notice that exercise - which is a key part of the structural pillar - strongly affects the other two. Aerobic exercise produces beneficial biochemical changes, which in turn improve our mental and emotional state. I experienced this dramatically during a very stressful time in my life. I had just gotten married, moved to a new city and was starting a new business with another couple. My stress was so intense that I became nauseous and found it difficult to eat. I was beside myself with worry and anxiety. Somehow I got into jogging for exercise. About 15-20 minutes into it, I could actually feel the stress drain out of my body as my mind and emotions cleared and I felt like myself again! Ever since then–and that was 1978–I have been a firm believer in exercise.

As another example of the interaction between pillars, consider the benefits of relaxation and meditation. Research has shown that as the mind and emotions calm down, our biochemistry also changes, lowering our blood pressure and pulse and balancing our stress hormones. Each pillar stands alone as a crucial aspect of our health, but all three are necessary to fully support excellent health and wellness. **It is valuable to consider that in this model we don't make one domain more important than another.** They are not placed in a top-down hierarchy with mental on top and physical on the bottom, as in many other healing systems. **All three domains are co-equal and provide a strong, balanced foundation or platform to support our healing and well being.** The good news is that improving a single area helps our entire being, and the bad news is that neglecting one area of life adversely affects the others. (This health model comes. from the founder of chiropractic, Dr. D.D. Palmer and is still the basis of chiropractic philosophy).

Excellent health is a question of balance and sometimes compromise. I often hear people say how "we all have to die sometime" as they are about to partake of their favorite indulgence. A key challenge is how to balance the joys of life with a sustainable lifestyle that incorporates disease prevention and health promotion. Too little joy and fun can harm us just as surely as that addiction to sugar. I have found it helpful to cultivate the joys of a healthy lifestyle and the energy and freedom which wellness brings. At this point in my life I feel blessed that most of the time I actually enjoy getting up early to do my morning routine of yoga, Tai Chi and meditation.

If you have a chronic or consistent health challenge, then by all means seek to find where your life is out of balance. Do you need to learn how to relax and find emotional healing? Are you out of shape and need to get moving? Or is building a better diet what you know you need to do? My recommendation is to pick one simple thing, as discussed in Chapter IV (question #4b. on worksheet), run the Wellness Process™ and get on with making it your new health habit. When that is secure, go on to the next item necessary to increase your health. The next three chapters provide many possible action steps (baby steps) for you to consider adding to your new wellness lifestyle.

Explaining the Boxes   **Baby Step #** □□□

*Throughout the rest of this book you will see, inside boxes, individual baby steps that are recommended and explained. My goal is to make them as user friendly and as understandable as possible! The baby steps will be numbered in order on the upper right of each text box and listed in the front of the book for cross-referencing. You will also see three small boxes after the number of each baby step. I suggest placing **one check** if you are mildly interested in considering taking the step, with no implied commitment. Place **two checks** if you are moderately interested, still with no commitment implied and **three checks** if you definitely want to commit to taking this baby step, despite any resistance!*

I suggest that you use the Wellness Process™ for any baby steps that you have checked three times and for which you have resistance! Just answer question #4b. with this baby step and proceed to answer the remaining questions.

CHAPTER IX
THE STRUCTURAL PILLAR

Exercise

This absolutely vital activity is composed of three main parts - cardiovascular or aerobic, stretching and strengthening. An ideal program will include all three in a unique proportion, depending on your needs. Cardio or aerobics has a direct and immediate beneficial effect on our heart, blood vessels and lungs. It also improves our mood and is a great anti-depressant. **For ideal body weight, healthy immune system and graceful aging, exercise is essential.**

If you are living a sedentary lifestyle, then walking may be the best all around exercise for you to start. All you need is a good pair of walking shoes or "cross trainers" and you are ready. Start wherever your tolerance allows and gradually increase your pace, duration and distance. A good rule-of-thumb is to work towards at least three to four days a week for 20-30 minutes, but the more the merrier. Other forms of aerobics include swimming, dancing, bike riding, jogging, aerobics classes, vigorous gardening or yard work, etc.

This type of exercise should be continuous and moderate, achieving a target pulse rate. This is computed by first subtracting your age from 220, then taking 70-80% of that. For instance mine would be 220-55 = 165 beats per minute and the target range would be 116-132. The less technical way of doing this is to exercise at a comfortable rate so that you are breathing deeply but still able to carry on a conversation. You should also be working up a mild sweat. For optimal benefit this target pulse should actually be sustained for a minimum of 15-20 minutes. Ideally the form or forms of exercise you choose should be fun and varied, something you can develop into a health habit and continue for the rest of your life. It is not so important what you do, as long as you do something on a regular basis. If you choose this as a Baby Step, then just make a commitment to yourself to get your cardio or aerobics at least three to four times per week and schedule it in!

Exercising Optimally   **Baby Step #1** ☐☐☐

Pick a suitable exercise (or exercises) that is interesting and appropriate for your level of fitness (or lack thereof). Set a goal for how many times per week and how long you want to do it. My minimum recommendation is 20-30 minutes, at least 3-4 times per week. Do it at a pace where you reach your aerobic threshold. Determine this either by working up a mild sweat and being slightly out of breath, or by achieving your target pulse rate as explained in the text above.

Stretching and strength training balance each other and are both necessary for a well-rounded program. Stretching is important to protect our muscles and joints and can be brief and simple or more elaborate, as in yoga. Ideally doing <u>some</u> stretching every day is beneficial. Strengthening is very important for our posture, preventing back and neck pain and staying ambulatory into old age. This involves exerting our muscles against resistance, as when using dumbbells, free weights or circuit training with machines. Every other day is ideal for this.

Stretching Program   **Baby Step #2** ☐☐☐

Begin to stretch on a regular basis. Develop your own routine to do at home or go to classes like yoga or the YMCA's Healthy Back Class. My minimum recommendation is 10-15 minutes per day 3-4 days per week. Good sources for stretches also include your chiropractor, physical therapist, trainer, yoga teacher, etc.

Strength and Power Building   **Baby Step #3**   ☐☐☐

This can be done at the gym using free weights or machines. Most gyms include a session or more with a trainer to get you started right. Some gyms are set up with a circuit, which is a series of machines that provides strength training for all your major muscle groups. If you go from machine to machine and don't rest between, then you can get an aerobic workout as well, while building strength. Strength training can also be done at home if you get free weights such as a barbell and/or dumbbells. My minimum recommendation is 20-30 minutes 3 times per week.

      Balance and agility are also important for physical fitness and can be increased with proper training. Tai Chi Chuan is excellent for doing this. I have experienced marked improvement in my balance from doing Tai Chi regularly. As we age, maintaining balance becomes crucial to prevent falling. If you are not interested in going to a Tai Chi class regularly or it is too big a step for you, then let me suggest a simple Tai Chi warm-up exercise. It is specifically good for balance and takes only about two minutes a day. The exercise is balancing on one foot. That's right! It may sound easy, but actually it can be quite challenging, depending on how you do it. Safety precautions to prevent falling are needed if you are elderly or have poor balance. Make sure you do this exercise next to a counter, sturdy table, desk or between two chairs (with their backs to you).

Exercising Balance   **Baby Step #4**   ☐☐☐

Bend your knees slightly and slowly raise one foot off the floor a few inches, or gradually all the way up, until your thigh is horizontal. You may also tuck the sole of your foot against your inner thigh as in the Tree pose of hatha yoga. Time yourself and see how long you can do it. You can use a watch, wall clock or just count seconds ("1-1000, 2-1000, 3-1000," etc.). Then switch legs. Your arms can be somewhat extended to improve your balance. When you are at the point where there is no challenge and you can easily hold steady 30 seconds or more, then do it with your eyes closed. Be prepared to lose your balance almost immediately! Vision is one of the three components of balance along with the vestibular (balance) sensors in the inner ears and proprioceptors (position and motion sensors) in the joints, muscles, tendons, etc. With practice you may be able to balance with your eyes closed for up to 30 seconds.

Balance exercises also play an important role in rehabilitation after injury and are helpful for all sports. Remember the importance of balance.

Posture

This aspect of health is an external reflection of our entire being. Posture develops and changes during our entire life and is both a cause and an effect. It affects our energy and comfort level, our organ function, our attitudes, the health of our joints and the likelihood of developing arthritis. Our posture also reflects our sitting, standing and habits of movement. Our attitudes, beliefs and childhood upbringing are all reflected in our posture as well. It can be improved slowly over time with increased awareness and by specifically stretching tight and shortened muscles and strengthening weak or flaccid ones. Poor posture increases our probability of back and neck pain, arthritis and digestive problems, to name just a few.

The positions or postures in which we sleep are also important. Generally, sleeping on our back and sides is good, but sleeping on our stomach can cause back and neck problems, though there are exceptions. Some people use a pillow under the knees while on their back and between the knees while lying on their side. Having just the right support under the neck is also very helpful.

Sculpting Posture   **Baby Step # 5** ☐☐☐

Here is a summary of ideas to evaluate and improve your posture:
1. Either on your own, or with professional help, rate your posture and decide which muscle groups need to be stretched and lengthened. Then decide which ones need to be toned through strengthening. Then do it!
2. Evaluate your sleep posture, the condition and suitability of your mattress and your pillow(s). How your muscles and joints feel

---

when you wake up is a good rule of thumb to determine overall need. Of course, there are other factors like diet and nutrition, stress level and quality of sleep. To have a good, supportive quality mattress is a blessing but the degree of firmness is a personal preference. For people with back problems, recent research indicates that a medium firm mattress may be better than a firm one! Your pillow should support your neck andgenerally keep your neck and head level with the rest of your spine, not too high or low.

3. If you are a stomach sleeper, then you can program yourself not to do that by wearing a shirt to bed with button-down pockets with a golf ball in each pocket. You will wake up every time you attempt to turn onto your stomach, thus breaking the habit within a few days!

4. Consider having an extra pillow to place under your knees when you are on your back, and between your knees when you are on your side.

Although sleeping itself is part of the mental domain, for convenience I will mention it here. Many folks in our society do not sleep enough and run up a **sleep debt**. This has destructive effects on our health, can diminish our mental function and make us accident-prone. Most adults need an average of 6-8 hours of sleep. This next baby step to health involves paying attention to how you feel after differing amounts of sleep and making an honest appraisal of what is optimum for you. Too much sleep is also detrimental. Once you have come up with the amount that works well for you, then make a point of getting that much on a regular basis. Be aware that your body needs more sleep when you are stressed or ill. Taking naps can also be very beneficial and is nothing of which to be ashamed. Although we have a cultural prejudice against it, many accomplished people take regular naps. To put a good spin on it I prefer to call it taking a *Power Nap*.

Sleep Time and Power Napping   **Baby Step #6** ☐☐☐

Monitor your mental clarity and rate of mistakes and accidents. Modify sleep time to maximize benefits and be willing to increase it during times of illness or high stress.

Consider taking *power naps* on a regular basis.

As Emerson once said, "Health is the first muse, and sleep is the condition to produce it."

Breathing

Although a physical activity, breathing has profound effects on our mental/emotional state and on our biochemistry. Whenever you can remember, stop what you are doing and take a few slow, deep breaths. This simple act induces relaxation, oxygenates and alkalizes the body, circulates lymph and other fluids and allows us to reflect and gain an expanded perspective. The way to get the most out of deep breathing is to inhale in three parts. This is called diaphragmatic breathing.

Deep Three-Part Breathing   **Baby Step #7** ☐☐☐

First place one hand over your belly just below your navel and the other over your chest, completely exhaling. Then as you start to inhale, preferably through your nose, allow your belly to expand, feeling your lower hand move out. This is done by relaxing the belly and then slightly pushing out. Next, allow your chest to expand, feeling your upper hand move out slightly. Finally, allow your shoulders to rise almost imperceptibly as you completely and comfortably fill your lungs. Pause for a moment and then let all the air out through your mouth with a sigh or slight "aah" or "haa" sound. Repeat three times and work up to ten repetitions.

If you spend some time doing breathing exercises then during the day even one conscious, slow deep breath will serve as an anchor, connecting you back to a more relaxed state.

Loving Touch

Under this topic I include hugging, physical affection, massage, bodywork and sexuality. Touch can actually be thought of as a nutrient, like vitamins or minerals, in that it is essential for our health. Like all mammals, we require loving touch and affection, especially as infants, for proper growth and development. Even as adults it is necessary for our health. I recommend at least three hugs per day. If you live alone or have recently ended an intimate relationship, then five or more are even better.

If you have never had a professional massage, then by all means find an experienced, licensed massage therapist and indulge yourself! You can ask friends or family for a referral or do a search on the American Massage Therapy Association website, www.amtamassage.org. The benefits of massage are enormous. They include decreased muscle tension and pain, as well as increased circulation, flexibility, range of motion and sense of well being.

Experiencing Massage   **Baby Step #8** ☐☐☐

This baby step is not only good for you, but it feels really good too. If you have never had a professional massage, then find a licensed massage therapist and schedule one. Consider getting a massage on a regular basis. My minimum recommendation is one to two per year and to maximize benefits, at least one to two per month.

An open secret among some women is the pleasure of receiving facials. They are wonderful for men, too. My wife is an esthetician (licensed facial technician), and I can tell you from personal experience that a facial is a very relaxing and nourishing experience! Of course it also beneficial for the health and appearance of the skin.

Sex and Wellness

Obviously there is much more to sex than just the physical release. Women are much more aware of this than men. I recommend looking into the study of Tantra or Sacred Sex to enhance this area of your life. Sexual function and our capacity for pleasure are both a reflection of our state of health and contribute to improving wellness.

Tantra involves the application of mindfulness to sexuality. Deep, slow, conscious breathing is used to prolong and deepen pleasure. It is essential that both partners are on the same page and that the channels of communication are open. See the section on relationships in Chapter IX, especially the two communication techniques, **Three Positives Before a Negative**, and the **Withhold Release**.

In Tantra for heterosexual couples emphasis is initially placed on the woman's pleasure. It is helpful for the woman to be open, receptive and trusting. As a woman, you can practice with your mate, asking for what you want, and being specific how and where you want to be touched. In practicing the exercise below, it is great to alternate roles so both partners get the experience. It is called the training cycle. My wife and I learned this from Ulla Angola, M.A. Check out her website at www.ullalcoaching.com.

The Training Cycle	**Baby Step #9** ☐☐☐

The first part involves asking your partner for a specific change in the way s/he is touching you. To simplify, focus on the three aspects of touch including (1) location, (2) pressure and (3) speed. Be specific and ask for a change of only one aspect at a time. For instance, "Could you please move a little slower?" Or, "Please use a bit more pressure." The second part involves giving positive feedback for any change before asking for additional changes. This way both partners get a win and the process energizes you. The whole thing would sound like this: "Honey, I love the way you are touching me right now and could you move your hand over to the left just a bit? Oh, that's great! Would you slow it down for me now? Wonderful! I really like that. How about just a bit less pressure? Perfect! Keep doing that, I love it!" In this way you and your partner don't have to be mind readers and you can be touched just the way you like.

For men, it is frequently recommended that the initial focus be on ejaculation control. This involves delaying orgasm, not having one every time you make love or separating ejaculation from orgasm. In Tantra the male partner shifts his focus from being goal oriented to being more present and playful with his partner. The focus is on the experience itself and on the exchange of "energy" between partners.

During intercourse, as pleasure builds, periodically stop moving well before the "point of no return," breathe deeply, then resume movement when the desire for orgasm has receded. Repeat this until both partners are satisfied.

Prolonging Pleasure　　　　　　　　**Baby Step #10**　□□□

A good technique for men to use initially to postpone orgasm and prolong pleasure is the mindful use of the breath and the cessation of all other movement. Pay attention to the whole body and use slow, deep breathing to draw the focus away from the genitals.

Performing Kegel Contractions　　　**Baby Step #11**　□□□

This is a great exercise for both sexes. It involves contracting the muscles of the pelvic floor and anus. It feels like lifting up and pulling in this area. These are the same muscles that are used to stop urination and this exercise can initially be practiced by consciously stopping the stream. Men can also use the kegel exercise during lovemaking to help delay orgasm and increase pleasure. For women, it is great to prevent prolapse or dropping of the bladder and uterus. It can be very pleasurable for both partners if the woman uses these muscles during intercourse to squeeze the male organ.

Have fun with these techniques and check out the following books: The Art of Sexual Ecstasy, by Margo Anand; Tantra, The Art of Conscious Loving, by Charles and Caroline Muir; and Mystical Sex, by Louis Meldman, Ph.D.

Hydrotherapy

This is a fancy way of saying the external use of water for health as opposed to drinking water, which is covered in Chapter IX, The Pillar of Biochemistry. Most cultures encourage using hot soaking baths for relaxation and improved circulation. You don't need an elaborate hot tub or Roman bath to soak in a nice warm bathtub. Women innately understand the value of this and bath more often than men. Even a shower can be used therapeutically by letting the hot water beat down on sore, tight shoulder and neck muscles. I also recommend contrast baths or hot and cold showers. You may need to go to a spa to alternate between a hot and cold tub, but anyone with a shower can get the same benefits at home. Alternating hot and cold is very relaxing and energizing at the same time, and stimulates the blood flow to the core (cold) and to the surface (heat). If the idea of a cold shower does not sound appealing to you, then I recommend that you experiment with the next baby step!

Contrast Showering   **Baby Step #12** ☐☐☐

Take your normal shower, except at the end lower the temperature just a bit until it feels cool. Let it flow over you, front and back, for a few moments until you long for the warmth again. Then go back to warm, but go slightly hotter than normal to the point where you actually desire (or are at least willing) to be cooled again. Then go back to cool, but try it slightly cooler than the first time. Try two to three cycles of this and, of course, level off on the hot so as not to scald yourself. With the cold cycle, the limit is straight cold, which can be quite cold in the winter.

I do this periodically all year round and our winter water in Ashland, Oregon, is melted snow from Mt. Ashland (8,000 feet). I personally find this technique very cool (pun intended)!

Physical Medicine
In illness, first look to the spine.
Hippocrates

Physical medicine is a natural form of health care that pre-dates the father of medicine, Hippocrates. Manipulation of the spine and joints has most likely been around since before recorded history, as the oldest Egyptian and Chinese manuscripts discuss its technique and virtues. Hippocrates wrote an entire treatise about it. In modern times, physical medicine is practiced primarily by physical therapists, some naturopaths, osteopaths and chiropractors. Chiropractors outnumber these other professions and perform the most spinal manipulations. **Chiropractic also has the most scientific and medical research confirming its effectiveness, cost-effectiveness and safety.** Chiropractors generally have more hours of training in school in manipulation than any other profession as well. A good resource for chiropractic information is the American Chiropractic Association website, www.amerchiro.org, which includes summaries of the scientific research done on chiropractic and provides help in finding a good chiropractor in your area.

Be aware that some M.D.s may have a negative opinion of chiropractic if they have only been exposed to the older, AMA (American Medical Association) propaganda. This has been slow to change since chiropractic won the anti-trust lawsuit against the AMA in 1987, which was upheld by the U.S. Court of Appeals in 1990 and finally upheld by the U.S. Supreme Court. Here is a summary of the Appeals Court decision*: (1) The AMA's illegal conspiracy to destroy the profession of chiropractic was pervasive. (2) Harm was done to the public by the AMA's illegal conspiracy as chiropractors were found to be more effective than medical doctors in certain segments of the health care market. (3) Harm was done to the chiropractic profession and to individual doctors of chiropractic. (4) The Court believed that the AMA could not be trusted to obey the law and that an injunction was necessary.*

"The times they are a changing" and chiropractic is becoming mainstream now. This is not only because it works well and people demand it, but also because of the extent of the valid medical and scientific research confirming this. The results that you get from manipulation depend on many things including the training, skill and experience of the practitioner. Look for a good match between your unique needs and what the practitioner offers. This includes not only getting effective pain relief, but leaving the office feeling straighter, taller and with an increased sense of well being. The philosophy and personality of the doctor or practitioner is also an important factor worth considering.

By all means, try chiropractic if you have not already done so (unless you are happy with the manipulation you are receiving from another type of practitioner). It may even be necessary to go to several different chiropractors until you find one who is effective for you. After all, how many different medical doctors have you seen in your life? If one does not help you that does not mean that you never see a medical doctor again. How many dentists have you seen? Isn't your physical body, with all its joints, complex spinal column and underlying nervous system worth being checked and tuned up or adjusted from time to time? I think so!

Another benefit of chiropractic is the recognition of the interaction between spinal structure and organ function. Obviously, not every condition can be cured through adjusting the spine, as some early chiropractors may have believed. However, there are many benefits to the entire body of having a well-tuned and highly functioning spine and nervous system. Research has even shown benefit to the immune system from spinal adjusting!

Finding a Chiropractor **Baby Step #13** ☐☐☐

To find a good chiropractor, start by asking local friends and relatives for a referral. Your primary care or family medical doctor may also know the best one for your particular needs. The American Chiropractic Association website (**www.amerchiro.org**) can help you find a good chiropractor in your area. You can check prices and determine if you have insurance coverage for chiropractic. You can also find out if you are restricted to certain practitioners and amount of treatment. Do not make your decision of who to see based solely on these considerations. Receive a series of chiropractic adjustments based on your individual needs and once you reach maximum benefit, consider receiving wellness or maintenance care.

Solving Chronic Pain

Sometimes after we have been injured, or experienced repetitive strain, we can be left with chronic joint and muscle pain. Often the cause of this is weakened, loose, or damaged ligaments, which haven't healed properly. Ligaments are the "straps" or cables that connect bone to bone and basically hold our bodies together. They allow our muscles to do their work of moving and stabilizing our joints. Tendons are the "sinews" that attach our muscles to our bones.

If we break a bone it is very painful initially but often heals quite well in a couple of months. When we sprain a joint, for example an ankle, shoulder or back, it is the ligaments that are primarily injured and this can take many months to heal. Unfortunately, some serious sprains never heal properly. This is one reason that doctors and therapists involved with physical medicine say that a "soft tissue injury" involving the ligaments can be more serious than a broken bone.

Consider this example. You are involved in a car accident, let's say you are rear-ended, which is the most common type. You go to the emergency room to get it checked out. You may have neck and back pain, headaches, pain between your shoulders and pain radiating down your arm or leg. After doing a physical exam and taking x-rays, you are told that "You are okay. There are no broken bones. You have *just* a neck and back strain and you should be fine in a few weeks. Here, just take these pills and see your doctor if you are not better." What is wrong with this picture? There is a significant chance that you may not heal for two to twelve months and may require extensive physical therapy, chiropractic care and rehabilitation. This injury can definitely be worse than a broken bone. As a matter of fact, some of these cases may never heal properly. The problem is often that scar tissue forms where the muscle and ligaments were injured, leaving the ligaments stretched and the joint unstable. This weakened joint tends to be re-injured more easily, causing chronic pain.

This is where prolotherapy comes in. If physical medicine, including chiropractic, deep tissue massage, physical therapy, rehabilitation and even acupuncture fail to return the area to normal, then I recommend the technique of prolotherapy be considered. This is a special therapeutic procedure performed by only a small group of specially trained medical doctors and osteopaths. It actually involves injecting small amounts of an irritant, usually sugar, into the weakened ligaments to stimulate them to go through the repair process. Over the years, I have referred many of my patients for prolotherapy with great success. After not healing completely from several accidents myself, I received a course of prolotherapy, which greatly helped my problems. These treatments are performed in my area by two excellent doctors, Carl Osborn, D.O. and Allen Thomashefsky, M.D. Go to their website, www.drtom.net, for a good article on the benefits of prolotherapy.

There are many other causes of chronic pain, however. If you suffer from one of them, then keep in mind the value of the wellness approach, in addition to working with traditional western medicine. Many "alternative therapies" like meditation, yoga, mild exercise, chiropractic and nutrition can make a significant difference in your pain level and in your attitude towards your pain. A useful and supportive book is, The Chronic Pain Solution, by James N. Dillard, M.D., D.C., C.Ac.

Solving Chronic Pain   **Baby Step #14** □□□

1. Work with alternative as well as traditional doctors in dealing with your pain challenge.
2. Do not underestimate the value of the wellness approach and use such techniques as meditation, yoga, chiropractic, massage, acupuncture and nutrition.
3. For chronic joint and muscle pain, locate a prolotherapy specialist in your area and obtain a consultation from them.

CHAPTER X
THE PILLAR OF BIOCHEMISTRY

Introduction

Nutrition is one of my favorite topics and is the centerpiece of this pillar. I started studying nutrition because of my own health problems in 1970. Having a minor in chemistry during my undergraduate work as a pre-med student and taking additional biochemistry for my Master's degree has enormously helped my understanding. During my four years of Chiropractic College I had three solid courses in nutrition. Since then I have taken numerous post-graduate courses, including a 100-hour certification in Clinical Nutrition. I also follow the medical literature concerning nutrition. Since 1982 I have integrated nutrition into my practice as a sub-specialty and helped many patients in this way.

Have you noticed now much confusion there seems to be about diet and nutrition in this country? The main reason for this is **NOT** that we don't know the truth. It is that **we have been "sold a bill of goods" by the huge commercial food processing industry** whose bottom line is making profit, not making us healthy. As a matter of fact, they have processed and manipulated the food supply so that most grocery store items are not only harmful to our health but are potentially addictive as well. Junk food is cool, glamorous and the norm. Sugars, bad fats, MSG, artificial colors and additives are used to deceive us. **It actually takes courage and much initial effort to swim against this torrent.**
Modern western (allopathic) medicine is complicit in this scheme as are certain parts of our government, including the Agriculture Dept. and the Food and Drug Administration (FDA).

I want to clearly distinguish between individual medical practitioners and organized medicine as represented by the American Medical Association (AMA). All of the medical doctors that I know personally are sincere, hard working people. Locally I have established an effective networking and referral relationship with many medical doctors, osteopaths and other specialists. We all work together for the benefit of the individual patient. My complaint is with the "medical establishment" which appears more concerned with keeping a stranglehold on the entire health care industry, than in helping people.

When it comes to nutrition and other forms of preventative and natural medicine, including chiropractic, the AMA is biased and along with the pharmaceutical industry influences what is and is not taught in medical schools. This has had a stifling effect on the understanding and interest of many medical doctors in these areas. Unfortunately, many M.D.s receive little or no training in nutrition and seem to carry the AMA's bias.

This tragic situation is further perpetuated by the pharmaceutical industry, whose goal is making money by selling drugs prescribed by doctors. The corporate owned mass media cooperates in this ruse as well. Good nutrition combined with preventative and alternative medicine is "bad for business", and the drug industry knows this. It would seem, the Food and Drug Administration, whose job it is to protect consumers, has been bought out by the big drug cartels to protect their profits instead.

You would think that it would be in the best interest of the insurance industry to support health and prevention. But for the most part, this is not so. Our nation's medical bill is well over 100 billion dollars yearly and is growing faster than inflation. The larger this total becomes, the more money traditional insurance companies can make by continually raising premiums. They always stay ahead of the curve and turn huge profits. This whole situation is similar to the tobacco industry, which knowingly manipulated nicotine levels to encourage addiction (and subsequent illness) in order to maximize profits. **The defacto objective of our food, drug, medical and insurance industries is to make enormous profits while keeping us sick and ignorant**.

We have to take matters into our own hands, become educated and make new choices. When it come to diet and nutrition, *I recommend that you actually become an expert in the needs of your own body, as no one else can do this better than you!* In the following sections, I have simplified this process for you by distilling years of research and experience into a few key principles. They can be implemented in a step-by-step fashion, like gradually increasing the weights at the gym. The Wellness Process™ will help you when you run into resistance. In effect, **I am giving you an all-purpose tool to make implementation easier along with a concise list of crucial steps to take.**

The familiar saying "You are what you eat." is cute but not exactly true. It should be something like, "You are what you can digest, absorb and assimilate." It is also important to be able to eliminate the waste products of digestion from your body. The issue is not just about our physical health. Your mood and consciousness are also affected. I would like to give a perfect example of this before we look at each individual building block of this pillar.

Let me call your attention to the destructive effects of excess sugar in the diet and the benefits of eating adequate protein at each meal. Eating simple or refined carbohydrates (sugars and white flour for instance) is like trying to put out a fire by throwing gasoline on it. Sugars are rapidly digested and absorbed causing an inflamatory reaction in our body and a spike in blood glucose. This sets off a hormonal cascade, first stimulating the release of insulin from the pancreas in the body's attempt to handle the glucose. Next, it triggers the release of stress hormones (adrenaline and cortisol) from the adrenal glands, which in turn can cause heart palpitations and the "symptoms" of low blood sugar. As this occurs over and over again the result is irritability and fatigue, weight gain, immune suppression and eventually, diabetes and heart disease. By replacing sugars with a balance of proteins, "good" fats and fiber-rich complex carbohydrates, we stabilize our blood sugar and hormones, feel energetic and relaxed, burn fat and prevent disease.

Water and Other Beverages

Most of us have heard the recommendation to drink at least 6-8 cups of water a day. The catch is how to do that and not feel bloated. Here's what you do: drink most of your water when your stomach is empty of food, about ½ to 1 hour before meals is ideal. That way it has passed through you and won't dilute your digestive juices, which can interfere with digestion. Drinking any beverage with meals interferes with digestion. That's right, **I recommend that you drink as little as possible with meals.** When not eating, water should be your main beverage followed by herbal and green tea and possibly diluted fruit juices. Soda pop, milk and undiluted juices are <u>NOT</u> recommended at any time.

Drinking Lots Of Water **Baby Step # 15** ☐☐☐

The challenge here is to drink at least 2 quarts (8 cups) of water each day and not dilute your digestive juices during meals. The solution is to drink 2-3 cups each time your stomach is the most empty of food. The ideal times for most people are first thing in the morning (at least 30 minutes before breakfast) and at least 30 minutes before other meals. If you do this three times a day you will ingest the recommended 2 quarts a day. Simple!

Research does point to some benefits of mild to moderate **alcohol** consumption, especially for the heart, but I don't recommend this because of the problems of liver disease and abuse. If you have a **soda pop** habit, kicking it should be a top priority. Diet drinks are probably even worse than sugar-sweetened drinks. The **Nutrasweet** or **Equal** that is used to artificially sweeten them is highly addictive, is a brain excitotoxin (irritates and excites brain cells to the point of death) and can cause many, many health problems. To help you get off soda pop, try diluting your favorite unsweetened fruit juice about 50/50 with sparkling water.

On Green Tea, Coffee and Caffeine

There is a lot of confusion out there about coffee. Fortunately the research is clear about a few things. Coffee is not good for you, especially more than one or two cups per day. It causes problems for the heart, stomach and pancreas. Decaffeinated coffee isn't really any better. Commercial decaffeination leaves toxic residues in the coffee and it still contains acids and other harmful chemicals. Green tea is good for you, despite the caffeine. It is a proven cancer-preventative, antioxidant and supports the stomach and liver. If you are good at logic, then you can deduce from the above that the problem is not the caffeine. It is the coffee itself that can cause health problems (however, caffeine can over-stimulate some people and interfere with sleep). If you are hooked on coffee, then switching to green tea makes it much easier to kick the habit.

Kicking The Coffee Habit	Baby Step #16 □□□

I have many patients who have successfully become coffee-free. This can be done by either gradually decreasing the dose or by going cold turkey. The gradual method works well by tapering off over several weeks and then just stopping. With the cold-turkey method you just stop. Either method can be facilitated by switching to green tea, which is a healthy source of smaller amounts of caffeine, without the toxins of coffee. The advantage of the sudden method is that you get it over with in about 4 days. The disadvantage is that you can get that famous coffee withdrawal headache often associated with fatigue. As mentioned above, green tea can help both the headache and the fatigue. Anyway you can quit, you will reap many health benefits and actually have more energy in the long run!

Diet

As mentioned in the introduction to this chapter, *diet can be a confusing topic because of all the vested interests working against our health.* In keeping with my theme of making wellness simple and attainable, **I want to present the most important and uncontroversial principles of eating for health.** Following all 5 of these principles may seem like a daunting task. If you want to improve your diet then remember to take "baby steps." I suggest you work with just one of these five principles at a time. They overlap, so by accomplishing just a few of them the rest will fall into place much more easily.

The Five Key Dietary Principles

❶ Eat a high proportion of unprocessed, natural and organic food.
❷ Eat and drink as little refined white sugar as possible.
❸ Eat balanced amounts of protein, carbohydrate and fat each meal.
❹ Eat "good" fats.
❺ Eat plenty of fresh vegetables every day, steamed and raw.

What follows is an explanation of these five principles presented as Baby Steps. Work with them in any way that seems best for you. I would like to suggest a possible strategy: start by increasing your consumption of vegetables (organic if possible) every day. This is probably the single most important change people most can make. Here's why: **As a group vegetables are the most nutrient rich foods, full of vitamins, minerals, phytochemicals and fiber.** They contribute to the prevention of virtually all chronic diseases. They act as one of the antidotes to sugar and junk food cravings. As a matter of fact, the opposite may also be true – if you are a junk food "addict" then you may have an initial aversion to eating vegetables. I strongly encourage you to get over this. Start by gradually finding a way to eat whatever vegetables you can, and eventually you will be able to kick the junk food habit and eat in a way that supports your health, wellness and higher values! Notice that just by eating more veggies, Principle #5, you also automatically increase your compliance of #1, # 2 and #3. *You will benefit from four out of the five principles with this one step. If you put a little extra virgin olive oil on your veggies and combine it with some "clean" protein, then you will be accomplishing all 5 steps!*

Eating Natural and Organic　　　　　**Baby Step # 17**　☐☐☐

Eat as high a proportion of unprocessed, natural and organic food as possible. An apple is better than apple juice, which is better than soda pop. Whole grain bread is better than "wheat" bread which is better than white bread. Free-range chicken is better than commercial factory chicken which is better than luncheon meat. Consider these changes as **upgrades** as in most cases both the nutritional content and the flavor are enhanced! *Unbiased scientific research has confirmed that most organically raised food does have superior nutritional value* and is worth the modest price increase. You do get what you pay for as well as supporting small family farms and the environment.

Minimizing the Use of White Sugar　　　**Baby Step #18**　☐☐☐

Eat and drink as little white refined sugar as possible. This follows from the previous baby step. The average consumption of sugar in this country is 165 lbs. per person per year. Everyone I know denies that they could possibly eat 1/3 lb. of sugar a day. Most of it comes in the form of "hidden sugar" occurring in processed foods. For instance, ketchup is mostly sugar on a caloric basis. **Read labels!!!** *I strongly recommend that you become a label reader.* There are many forms of refined sugar being added to processed foods and labels are required to list ingredients in order of quantity. Look out for sucrose, fructose, dextrose and high fructose corn sweetener, to name a few. Raw sugar, succanat and brown sugar are mostly just plain sugar. Artificial sweeteners may be worse than sugar, especially Equal or Nutrasweet, for which the FDA has received more complaints than any other food additive. Leave it alone! Honey is twice as sweet as regular sugar, has some good properties and is O.K. if used very sparingly. Maple, rice and fruit syrup and date sugar can also be used very sparingly. Are there any good sweeteners? Not really, with two notable exceptions – the medicinal sugar **xylitol** and the herbal extract **stevia**. Xylitol looks and tastes like regular sugar but does not trigger a harmful insulin response and it actually inhibits bacteria in the mouth, helping to prevent dental cavities and ear infections. Stevia is a great herbal sweetener, has no calories and may actually be beneficial. So go ahead and **get to know** <u>xylitol</u> **and** <u>stevia</u> **and kick the sugar habit!**

Balancing Proteins, Carbohydrates and Fats   **Baby Step #19** ☐☐☐

Eat a balanced amount of protein, carbohydrate and fat at every meal. One of the biggest problems I see is excessive consumption of carbohydrates like bread, bagels, crackers, chips, potatoes, rice, pasta, cookies, pastries, sweets, soda pop, etc. Eat only a modest amount of unrefined carbs at each meal or snack and think of balancing it with a protein and good fat (see below). A moderate portion of carbohydrate would be one slice of whole grain bread or ½ bagel, or a cup of cooked brown rice, or a small portion of pasta, or a small baked potato. Also include a moderate amount of ***clean protein*** (free range, humanely slaughtered, organic, non-farmed[fish], without nitrates, pesticides, hormones or antibiotics) at each meal. *Breakfast seems to be the most difficult for some people. Who says it has to be cold cereal, coffee and* *juice?* It can be like a small lunch or dinner with clean protein, unrefined carbohydrate, vegetables and good fat!

If you like eggs consider having three for breakfast but discard 1 or 2 of the yolks to keep the fat moderate. The Zone Diet, by Barry Sears, Ph.D., presents a good rule of thumb by having a 40-30-30 ratio of carbohydrate to protein to fat. Another diet program I like is The Omega Diet, by Artemis Simopoulos, M.D., that emphasizes the importance of increasing the beneficial Omega 3 oils in our diet. Also helpful is the book Syndrome X, by Burton Berkson and Jack Challem, which is especially good for reducing carbohydrate addiction and preventing diabetes. The Schwarzbein Principle, by Diana Schwarzbein, M.D., has a similar approach, and there are other good sources for further reading. If you are overweight and eat a lot of carbohydrates, then you may need stronger measures. There is a great probability that you are actually addicted to these carbs. Unless you break free, your health will severely suffer and you may never be able to permanently lose weight. You may need to go on a reduced carbohydrate diet originally made popular by Dr. Atkins but greatly modified so as not to jeopardize your overall health and wellness. (See the section on Permanent Weight Loss.)

Eating "Good" Fats   **Baby Step #20** ☐☐☐

Eat essential, or good fats occur in nuts and seeds, beans, whole grains, fish and flax. *The idea of eating low fat is a myth,* based largely on misunderstanding. Eating the common commercial forms of fats and oils can be deadly, however. Corn, safflower and peanut oils contain an overabundance of Omega 6 oils and are harmful in excess. The jury is still out on canola oil. Processing, frying or cooking most oils creates harmful trans fats. These are oils that actually have their chemical shape altered and they wreck havoc in the body, including raising cholesterol levels. This is why margarine is so harmful and butter is better. An even bigger shocker is that pure coconut oil **IS** good for you and great for cooking. (We have been mislead by the Agriculture Dept. is support of domestic oils).

Cold water, fatty fish is the best source of Omega 3. **If you don't eat fish, then it is essential that you get your Omega 3s**

elsewhere. Flax, hemp and walnuts are good vegetarian sources. Olive oil is the best all-around oil because it is very stable and balanced, containing oleic acid, which is an Omega 9 oil. It can be used for cooking without breaking down and forming trans fats. It is also low in Omega 6, of which most of us have an excess. Consider adding up to 4 tbsp. of ground-up flax seeds to your diet, starting with one tbsp. and working up to 4. This is best done by getting a coffee grinder just for flax, and grinding it fresh every day or so. Sprinkle on foods or make a paste by adding a little water and stevia to sweeten to taste. Not only will this add fiber and Omega 3 to your diet, but flax seeds also contain lignans, which are phytochemicals that help prevent cancer, especially breast, colon and prostate.

Eating Lots Of Vegies   **Baby Step #21** ☐☐☐

Eat lots of fresh (organic) vegetables every day, steamed and raw in salad. In my opinion, eating more vegetables is probably the single most important improvement you can make to your diet. This does not include starchy vegetables such as corn and potatoes. Fruit can be overeaten as well. Most people would benefit from eating one to two pieces of fruit a day, but more than that can exceed the tolerance for carbohydrates. By the way, berries are fabulously nutritious and a good-sized handful only counts as one piece of fruit. Along with flax, *the single best thing most people can do to improve their diet and health is to eat at least one cup of steamed leafy green vegetables every day* (this would be 2-3 cups of raw greens before cooking). This includes Swiss chard, spinach, kale, collards, mustard, bok choy, beet tops, etc. Not only are they high in vitamins, minerals, chlorophyll and fiber, but they also are high in anti-cancer phytochemicals. So Mama was right, "Eat your veggies!"

Nutritional Supplements

It is important to remember that supplements are just that, supplements. They are not meant to replace a good diet. For basically healthy people, supplements act as a type of health insurance and can fill in and round out any borderline deficiencies in the essential vitamins and minerals. **Research has shown that the vast majority of Americans are actually deficient in one or more major essential nutrient!** This is one reason the Standard American Diet is **S.A.D**. If you are sick or suffer from a chronic illness, supplementation can also be a therapeutic part of your treatment plan. For a specific and individually tailored supplemental program, see a specially trained naturopath, chiropractor or holistic medical doctor.

This is more important than ever as our soils are becoming tragically depleted, primarily because of agribusiness practices. Artificial fertilizers only replace a few of the needed minerals and compost is rarely used. Pesticides also create imbalances in plants and soils. The net result is that plants look good but are low in nutritional value and high in toxic residues.

For general good health and disease prevention, I recommend a comprehensive, high potency multi-vitamin/mineral and extra vitamin C. Usually one-a-day tablets are **NOT** good, as they are low potency, incomplete and compressed too hard during manufacturing for good absorption. The best kind of multi is usually in capsules and designed to be taken 3-6 a day, since fitting in all the essential nutrients in significant doses takes up a lot of space. In addition, a calcium complex is a good idea, especially for women and should include magnesium, vitamin D, vitamin K and boron. The carbonated form of calcium is the cheapest but poorest in absorption. The best readily available forms are Citrate, Citrate-Malate, and Hydroxyapatite. Calcium is best taken morning and evening with food, as it needs stomach acid for best absorption. Milk may not be a good source of calcium as it may hinder absorption. **Cow's milk is great for calves but not for adult humans and is not recommended!**

In addition to the above supplements, consider taking a good fish oil or flaxseed oil supplement if you don't eat fish or flax seeds regularly. If you can't seem to get enough veggies down, then consider a green drink mix containing dried vegetables, grass juices, seaweeds, herbs and green algae (including spirulina and chlorella.) Grape seed extract is an excellent all-around phytochemical that is a powerful antioxidant and beneficial for the circulatory system. Glucosamine sulphate has strong scientific evidence supporting its use for arthritis and cartilage degeneration. Saw Palmetto also has impressive research supporting its use for enlarged prostate (benign prostatic hypertrophy,

BPH). There actually are hundreds of herbs that have been proven safe and therapeutically effective!

I have recently learned about an extract from the herb called *Chaparral* or *Larrea*. It has many valuable uses including that of antioxidant and natural anti-inflammatory, but its anti-viral effects particularly impress me. **It is a "slam-dunk" for herpes and shingles**, two very annoying and extremely painful conditions. I want to get the word out about this and recommend the website **www.larreamed.org** to obtain accurate information about this herb. It has been called "the mother of all plants" (Shegoi) by Native Americans and their "medicine chest." I have become an independent distributor of this product because I have seen it bring relief to many sufferers of herpes and shingles. *There is good medical research confirming its safety and its superior effectiveness for these two conditions compared to other products on the market, including prescriptions.* You can find out how to order it directly by calling 1-877-536-4716.

If you are not taking any supplements, then adding a good quality multi or even just 500 to 1000 mg. of vitamin C once or twice a day would make an effective Baby Step!

Supplementing For Health   **Baby Step #22** ☐☐☐

If you are not currently taking nutritional supplements then I recommend that you start. If you are already taking them, great, then I recommend that you evaluate what you are taking in light of the section above. Start with either a good quality, high potency comprehensive multi vitamin/mineral or 500-1000 mg. of vitamin C once or twice per day. Once you have gotten off to a good start with one, then add in the other, or just start off with both if that seems reasonable for you. In order of priority, consider adding the following supplements as you master the previous steps:
1. A highly absorbable calcium complex twice a day with breakfast and dinner
2. Flaxseeds (3-4 rounded tbsp daily) or flaxseed oil (2-3 tbsp per day) if you are a vegetarian. Use purified pharmaceutical grade fish oil (1-2 tsp a day depending on concentration) if you are not a vegetarian
3. Other supplements as need and interest dictate

A Word About Enzymes

Enzymes are chemical catalysts produced within the body. They facilitate all the biochemical reactions in the body and are ultimately under control of our DNA. In practical terms, there are two main categories of enzymes, digestive and systemic. As the name implies, digestive enzymes are involved in digesting our food, both in the stomach and small intestine. Systemic enzymes do their work inside every cell throughout the body and are responsible for just about all the other chemical processes in the body. They in turn are regulated by hormones and other chemical messengers from our DNA. The effectiveness of both types of enzymes are crucial to our good health.

In the stomach, the main digestive enzyme produced is pepsin, which needs an acid medium to start protein digestion. This underscores the importance of having a proper level of stomach acid (see next section on Digestion). As partially digested food moves along to the small intestine, its acidity also acts as a stimulus for the digestive juices to be released. Many digestive enzymes come into play here and are necessary for digesting carbohydrates, fats and proteins. This phase of digestion requires an alkali or basic environment, so all the stomach acid must be neutralized. The enzyme lactase is released here, which is necessary for breaking down milk sugar, or lactose. The deficiency of this enzyme is a genetic trait and is responsible for lactose-intolerance.

Therapeutically, digestive enzymes can be taken as supplements, both with food and on an empty stomach. When taken with meals they can help improve digestion. These include bromelain from pineapple stems and papain from papaya, which help break down protein. Other "plant enzymes" are available to help digest a broad spectrum of food constituents. Traditionally supplemental enzymes are obtained from the pancreas of animals. Enzymes can also be taken on an empty stomach, which allows some of them to be absorbed and utilized throughout the body. The most research has been done on protein digesting (proteolytic) enzymes. Bromelain and the pancreatic enzyme chymotrypsin are very effective when taken between meals. They have anti-inflammatory effects throughout the body, help to relieve pain, swelling, trauma, lessen allergic reactions and even decrease the viscosity of mucus. In addition bromelain is known to enhance the effects of other drugs, particularly antibiotics when taken for sinus and respiratory infections.

Raw food advocates correctly point out that cooking breaks down enzymes in food. However, this may not be such a great loss. The enzymes in most foods are not important to the body as far as I can tell from the scientific research done so far. There are many other benefits of eating some of our food raw, however. This includes reducing the problems of over cooking, frying or browning food. When carbohydrate foods are cooked this way, for example chips and french fries, the known carcinogen, acrylamide, is produced. It is currently being studied to determine the magnitude of the danger. Overheating or browning protein foods like meat, fish and chicken produces other carcinogens called heterocyclic amides. Barbecuing food produces the highest level of these compounds (darn!). Other benefits of eating some food raw is simply that the foods eaten this way are mostly fruits and vegetables. The benefits of these foods include high levels of vitamins, minerals, fiber and especially phytochemicals. For the most part, these benefits are not lost through cooking. So do eat a certain percentage of your food raw (approximately 20-30%), avoid overheating and browning food and consider enzyme supplementation.

Eating Raw Food and Enzymes **Baby Step # 23** □□□

1. Eat a certain percentage of your food raw. Experiment with this ratio and try varying it throughout the year, more in summer and less in winter.
2. Avoid overheating, frying, or excessively browning foods.
3. Consider taking digestive enzymes with meals if needed (see the next section on digestion).
4. Also consider supplementing with enzymes between meals for their systemic benefits, including relief from pain, trauma, bruising and swelling.

Digestion

Good digestion starts with creating a relaxed atmosphere around eating and chewing your food well. There is an old saying, "Chew your liquids and drink your food." This means chew solids so well that your food is liquefied before you swallow and swallow liquids slowly, one small mouthful at a time. Another health tip instructs us to chew each mouthful of food 100 times. These health aphorisms may be an exaggeration, but there is a kernel of truth in them.

Simplifying the way food groups are combined supports digestion. Most systems of food combining are overly complex and do not take individual differences into account. If you feel uncomfortable after eating or burp up and taste certain foods or certain combinations of foods, chances they aren't being digested well. Personally I have found that fruits don't combine well with vegetables or proteins, especially raisins and other dried fruits (which can produce a lot of intestinal gas.) Melons are best eaten alone. Vegetables go well with protein or carbohydrates, but large portions of both protein and carbohydrate don't mix well for many people. Of course large portions of carbohydrate are not recommended anyway because they are converted to sugar and over stimulate insulin production. **Experiment for yourself and see what works best for your unique biochemistry.**

When food reaches the stomach we need to produce a significant amount of stomach acid. As we age, less and less stomach acid is produced. Many people who suffer from the type of indigestion called heartburn or acid reflux actually have a deficiency of stomach acid (HCl). Yes, this is counter-intuitive and often the opposite of what many doctors say, as well as those ads touting antacids for relief of heartburn. The acid in a healthy stomach after eating should be as strong as battery acid (Ph 1-2). This is necessary for proper digestion in the stomach and it also serves as the trigger to the small intestine to release its digestive juices. That burning feeling that antacids only temporarily relieve is usually caused by an "unhappy" stomach. This means that when the stomach is irritated and/or low in acid it tends to regurgitate up some of its contents, which are still acid enough to burn, but not acid enough to properly digest food and keep the stomach "happy." **Reflux or burping up usually means the stomach is actually low in acid.** By eating properly with smart food combining you can usually prevent heartburn and reflux. Sometimes supplementing with HCl (stomach acid) with Pepsin is necessary and this should be done under the direction of a nutritionally oriented health professional. This is necessary because if you actually have an ulcer then HCl is contra-indicated and in this case can cause burning.

Stomach ulcers do need to be treated in a different matter. Here, too, it is usually not excess acid but the presence of harmful bacteria called H. pylori that weakens the stomach lining. Most ulcers are successfully treated now by killing these bacteria. **Ask your doctor to test for H. pylori if you have an ulcer.**

Other aids to digestion include taking digestive enzymes and/or beneficial bacteria like Lactobacillus acidophilus. Following the five basic principles in the diet section will insure you are getting enough fiber for your system. Remember to drink a lot of water but **not** with meals!

For more serious and chronic conditions of the bowel, I suggest you find a practitioner who utilizes the 4R® (registered trademark of Metagenics) gut restoration program as developed by Jeff Bland, Ph.D., founder of the Institute of Functional Medicine. Dr. Bland is a world renown expert in the field of nutritional biochemistry.

The 4 Rs stand for:

Remove	— pathogens, parasites and food allergies
Replace	— missing stomach acid and enzymes
Repair	— damaged, inflamed and leaky gut lining
Re-inoculate	— with beneficial bacteria

This is the most comprehensive program I have found for improving digestion and overall health. The UltraClear line of products were developed by Dr. Bland and are marketed by Metagenics, the largest supplement supplier to professionals. Dr. Bland is now the president and chief science officer of Metagenics.

Enhancing Digestion   **Baby Step #24**   □□□

1. First assess your level of need by the severity of symptoms and feedback from your doctor.
2. Start simplifying your diet by applying the basic principles of food combining and good nutrition described in this chapter.
3. Consider adding a good quality, highly viable acidophilus product to your supplement program. Experiment with adding a good digestive enzyme with each meal.
4. Read the section on *hidden food allergies* later in this chapter. If you have any chronic symptoms please consider testing - by temporarily eliminating from the diet - a few likely suspects, especially wheat and dairy products.
5. If you do not find relief from the above steps then search out a qualified health care professional versed in this area. You can start by looking for a referral from Metagenics or from the Institute of Functional Medicine listed in the resource section in Part III.

Cleansing and Detoxification: Spring Clean Your Body!

      Good digestion and detoxification go hand in hand. By detox we mean the ability of the body to neutralize and eliminate poisons or toxins. These substances are produced within the body or enter from the environment. Alcohol and drug detox (rehab) is a related but different process than the one discussed here.

      Toxins are produced within the body by normal metabolism and by abnormal processes as well. An example of an abnormal process is the waste products produced by unfriendly or harmful bacteria or yeast (Candida) in the gut or colon. This can become a source of serious health problems manifesting as headaches, fatigue, skin problems, indigestion, fibromyalgia, some forms of arthritis, recurrent infections, premature aging, etc. This buildup of toxins becomes more serious as the colon wall is irritated and becomes more porous, leaking toxins directly into the system—called leaky gut syndrome.

The liver is the next organ in line affected by this problem. The body is designed to handle a certain amount of toxic material, as all the blood from the colon drains directly to the liver. One of the liver's main jobs is to neutralize and detoxify these poisons. All the blood in your system passes through the liver many times daily. The kidneys "merely" filter out the toxins after the liver has processed and neutralized them. **The liver's main job is like a chemical factory and a sewage treatment plant combined!**

It is crucial that you understand this, as the liver is perhaps the most overworked organ in the body. Why is this so important? Every single one of us living in the 21st century is being exposed to literally thousands of synthetic chemicals, hundreds of which are known to cause cancer, birth defects, sterility and auto-immune disease. This may be of greater concern than even heart disease, which is leveling off in this country, though it is still the number one cause of death.

The incidence of some forms of cancer is increasing in epidemic proportions. *Learn to protect your body from this environmental onslaught, or you too, could become a cancer statistic.* **Learn to live a lifestyle that prevents cancer**. This can't be emphasized enough! I have chosen this for myself, for my family and I recommend it to everyone with whom I come in contact. Once this dreaded diagnosis is made, the treatment of cancer is a long, painful and heroic journey, often unsuccessful. Please take this to heart. Do everything within reason to live a lifestyle that prevents cancer in the first place. True, some forms of cancer have a genetic tendency to occur, but the vast majority are environmentally and lifestyle related. The point is, modifying your lifestyle is attainable as opposed to trying to change your genes! By all means, educate yourself. There are many good books, organizations and websites available to help you. Re-dedicate yourself to this wellness journey.

If you find this information stressful then stop, take a deep breath, and be willing to re-evaluate your lifestyle and to prioritize! *Knowledge is power and ignorance is suffering.* Don't stick your head in the sand and deny what is happening, but be grateful that we now have the understanding and methods to prevent most forms of cancer.

The key is to periodically detoxify the body by supporting liver function and the digestive process. I recommend the use of Dr. Bland's UltraClear products under the direction of an experienced health professional. Following the recommendations in the Diet, Supplement and Digestion sections is the foundation for any successful detox program. **Develop a health-building diet that you can live with and enjoy.** The statement, "Diets don't work," is true in that the best way for you to eat is consciously with sustainable choices and not by playing the yo-yo game. That is, repeatedly crash dieting to lose weight only to gain it back. From a place of eating an enjoyable and satisfying health-building diet, then *you can periodically do cleansing and detoxification.* I recommend taking the self-scoring quiz, the Medical Symptoms Questionnaire (MSQ) that you will find in Appendix B where I have also included the Modified Elimination Diet.

Most traditional forms of fasting for detox have been found to be less than ideal because of the lack of certain nutrients including amino acids from protein. It has been discovered that the main detox pathways are in the liver and they need specific vitamins, minerals and amino acids to function. *A better approach than fasting has been developed and is called the Modified Elimination Diet.* **This has the benefits of fasting without starving.** This scientifically tested and proven cleansing diet avoids the danger of suppressing liver function and of losing muscle mass.

Yo-yo dieting and fasting cause a loss of healthy muscle tissue. Muscle is crucial to our health, fitness and is essential for actually burning fat. So not only is fasting and yo-yo dieting bad for detoxification, but also harmful for weight loss. The Modified Elimination Diet involves eating clean, healthy foods that are low in allergens. It emphasizes organic foods including vegetables and some fruit, free-range fowl, non-farmed fish, legumes and non-gluten grains. It can be combined with a partial meal replacement supplement or medical food which contains antioxidants, natural anti-inflammatories and detox factors to support liver, kidney and intestinal function.

After reading the next section on allergies, if you want to do a cleanse, then I suggest you follow Baby Step #25, which combines the Modified Elimination Diet with food allergy detection and elimination.

Hidden Food Allergies

Allergies are often a confusing and frustrating condition. Most people are familiar with the immediate type allergic reactions to substances like peanuts, strawberries and bee venom. These can be serious, even life threatening, but are usually well managed medically. Hay fever (pollen allergy) and other inhalant allergies to dust and molds are caused by the same mechanism and are technically called **Immediate Hypersensitivity Reactions**. *There is another type of allergy that is less recognized but much more common – some would say a hidden epidemic.* I am speaking of hidden food allergies or, technically, **Delayed Hypersensitivity Reactions**. These insidious reactions are slow to develop and are triggered by some of the most commonly eaten foods like wheat, dairy, egg, soy, corn, yeast, nuts, oranges, coffee and chocolate. That's right! These are the "foods of commerce" that most of us eat several times a day. Fortunately, not everyone has a problem with them.   However**, 50% or more of people with chronic health problems have hidden food allergies** and do react adversely to one or more these foods. Some of the most common health conditions they affect include headaches, irritability, depression, joint and muscle pain, frequent infections, arthritis, skin problems, digestive problems, migraines, IBS (irritable bowel syndrome), fibromyalgia and chronic fatigue.

To make the situation worse, *we can actually become addicted to the foods to which we are allergic*. The reactions to these foods are mostly unrecognized. They may not show up for 24 hours or more and, if eaten every day, can contribute to the ongoing, chronic conditions mentioned above. Each time we consume these foods though, the body undergoes a stress reaction, culminating in the release of endorphins, the body's own opium-like pain relievers. This is what we become addicted to, and thus, we actually feel worse without the allergic food and eventually we crave it. As with other addictions, there is a tendency to increase the dose or portion. This can then produce weight gain and binging. **Often the food eaten during a binge is a food allergy that has become an addiction.**

Is there a way out? Unlike immediate allergies, which usually show up on the well-known skin or patch test, these hidden allergies are hard to test for and only show up on a special blood test. **There is another practical method of identifying hidden food allergies that is inexpensive and reliable.** It is called Elimination/Provocation, which means that the suspected food is taken out of the diet for at least 4 to 14 days, symptoms are carefully monitored, and then the food is re-introduced again as symptoms continue to be monitored. If you feel better and find some relief without the food and feel worse when it is introduced, then you have successfully identified a culprit or allergen. Some allergens are fixed and must be avoided for life, like gluten (found in wheat and some other grains) for patients with celiac disease. Other allergens can be retested or may sometimes eaten sparingly on a rotational basis, usually once every 4-7 days. Of course you can choose to ignore it, but then you must face the consequences.

Alternatively, foods can be eliminated and tested one at a time. The next Baby Step explains how you can test all the common allergens at the same time combined with The Modified Elimination Diet and get the benefits of fasting while still eating (see Cleansing and Detoxification Section.) <u>Usually after one to three weeks there is a marked improvement in how you feel and then one suspected food is eaten to test it each day.</u> Within a week or so most of the common food allergies can be tested this way. Your unique health-building diet can then be constructed through eliminating the offending foods and by applying the 5 Key Principles from the Diet Section. This may sound like a lot of work, but if your health is suffering and/or you are serious about disease prevention and wellness, it is well worth the effort and will produce a lifetime of benefits. Remember, *ignorance is suffering and knowledge is power!*

This technique uses your own body as a laboratory to find out which foods work and which ones don't work for your unique biochemistry. It takes a lot of the guesswork and confusion out of eating for health. As I tell my patients during this process, it calls upon a mature perspective; a small short-term loss (giving up some comfort foods) for a long-term gain (discovering which foods work best for a lifetime of health and wellness). Continuing to eat according to cravings and binging in the face of chronic health problems and excess weight represents an immature perspective; a short-term gain for a long-term loss. *There is a better way !*

Allergy-Free Cleansing   **Baby Step#25** □□□

To help determine how badly you need this step, take the Medical Symptoms Questionaire (see Appendix B) and add up your score.

    0-25   Modest need, 7-10 days recommended
    26-50   Moderate need, 2 weeks recommended
    51-75   Moderately high need, 3 weeks, consider professional
            supervision
    76-100 High need, 3-4 weeks plus supervision from health
            professional strongly advised
    100+   Extreme need, four weeks or more, must work with a
            professional

(These ranges are approximations and the recommendations are based on my own clinical experience) Take the survey at weekly intervals and watch your score drop. The higher the score, the more room for improvement. In my four week cleansing groups (*The Great Ashland Detox*) I have frequently seen over 75% reductions in score. Even a 50% drop makes a huge difference in how you feel and in disease prevention. Also, the higher your initial score, the greater likelihood you may experience short-term discomfort or aggravation of your symptoms. This has been called a "healing crisis" and is minimized by following the program properly. It is commonly experienced as mild and brief flu-like symptoms such as fatigue, body aches and headache. This is one reason that the higher your initial score, the more likely you will need professional guidance including tailored nutritional support.

The basic program is to follow the Modified Elimination Diet for as long as recommended. Then re-introduce the common allergic foods one day at a time until they have all been tested. If you do get a reaction from a food, eliminate it from your diet, make careful note of it and wait an extra day or two until symptoms clear before testing the next food.

The advanced form of the program involves using one of the UltraClear products as a partial meal replacement and working with a health professional familiar with their use.

Hormones — The Good, The Bad and The Ugly

This is another important topic, which is potentially confusing and controversial. There is also a lot of disinformation that has been disseminated by the drug companies and unfortunately repeated by many well-meaning doctors. Let's look at how we can clarify this situation and give you some simple positive actions to take.

Estrogen and Progesterone

A woman has three main forms of estrogen in her body that are essential for health. These hormones start to decline at least 5-10 years preceding menopause. Menopause is usually defined as going six months to a year without a period. The emotional changes can often severely challenge a woman's life and family. It can also stimulate tremendous emotional growth and increase authenticity. Standard medical practice has been to prescribe artificial estrogen and related progestins to help with the symptoms, especially hot flashes, and presumably to slow or retard bone loss. This has proven to be a fiasco, as large recent studies have shown little benefits and serious increased risks of cancer, stroke and heart disease. It seems that the main benefit of this potentially dangerous drug, extracted from pregnant mare's urine (hence the trade name Premarin) has been to enrich the drug company's coffers. This is where it gets ugly. Apparently the drug companies had known this for years from earlier studies and continued to market these drugs to all menopausal women. As one claim after another was disputed, they would come up with another one and market it in such a way as to produce an emotional attachment or addiction in women and their doctors. This was done by touting the use of estrogen as being able to create a state of "feminine forever." See the book, <u>The Greatest Experiment Ever Performed On Women</u>, by Barbara Seaman. Once again this is a similar strategy to that used by the junk food industry and by the tobacco industry (who continued to market cigarettes even while denying knowledge of the cancer risks and also adjusting the nicotine and other additives to make the most addictive product possible).

Many women are switching successfully to herbs and other supplements as well as natural, bio-identical forms of estrogen and progesterone. Natural progesterone, as opposed to synthetic progestins (such as Provera) is often helpful for PMS and the early stages of menopause called peri-menopause (the years before menses stop completely). A combination of natural, bio-identical estrogens and progesterone is helping many menopausal women feel better and may also prevent bone loss without the side effects. Further testing needs to be done.

Lifestyle factors that women can incorporate include the five key dietary principles mentioned earlier. *Because estrogen balance depends on healthy liver and intestinal functions, supporting these organs is essential.* Decreasing or eliminating alcohol and alternating detoxification with a health-building diet supports the liver. More fiber and a good acidophilus supplement specifically helps balance estrogen by way of the intestines. Bone health is supported by weight-bearing exercise and by decreasing or eliminating alcohol, coffee and smoking. Your supplementation should include a highly absorbable form of calcium with magnesium, vitamin D and K, and the trace mineral boron.

Heart disease is another risk which increases for women after menopause and, here again, a wellness lifestyle has been shown to be your first line of defense. Fortunately, these are the same lifestyle recommendations as mentioned above. In addition, eating an Omega 3 rich diet and/or supplementing with purified fish oil and/or flax helps both your bones and your heart. Remember that if you choose to implement this program take one manageable Baby Step at a time. I recommend working with a health professional versed in these matters and also getting a copy of Dr. Christine Northrup's book, The Wisdom of Menopause.

Safe Passage Through Menopause   **Baby Step #26** ☐☐☐

Get a copy of The Wisdom Of Menopause. Read it, apply what it says and find a compatible health care professional with whom you can work.

Testosterone

This is the key hormone of masculinity and even women need a little bit for their libido and bone health. It has gotten a bum rap because young male body builders were taking large doses of the synthetic form of the hormone and suffering severe health consequences. Natural testosterone can be used safely and effectively by older men (40 and up) to prevent or reverse the negative effects of the male version of menopause, called ***andropause***. Symptoms are often assumed to be the natural consequences of aging and are ignored. They include weight gain around the belly, loss of strength, libido, inspiration, creativity, etc., and increased risk of heart disease. Testosterone has also been blamed for prostate cancer, but it does not <u>cause</u> it. If prostate cancer pre-exists then even natural testosterone supplementation can stimulate its growth and must be avoided.

To maintain wellness during andropause (male menopause) lifestyle factors are essential. Eat according to the Five Key Principles as stated in the diet section of this chapter and get sufficient aerobic exercise. As men age, our bodies actually start to produce more estrogen and our testosterone level drops. The key for aging men is to keep this ratio in balance. The five fundamentals for men to age well are: (1) getting and keeping body fat normal, especially belly fat; (2) decreasing or eliminating alcohol consumption; (3) detoxifying and supporting liver function; (4) supplementing with zinc in the range of 60-90 mg. a day depending on need; and (5) staying actively engaged in life, emotionally, mentally and spiritually! In addition, there are other supplements, including herbs and hormone precursors, that are available without a prescription.

Beyond this, you definitely need a knowledgeable health care professional to order blood tests and possibly prescribe natural forms of testosterone. A great resource for this whole topic can be found on the Life Extension website (www.lef.org under Protocols: Male Hormone Modulation Therapy).

The Challenges of Andropause   **Baby Step #27** ☐☐☐

This action step involves a two-fold challenge. The first is for aging men **to acknowledge** they are going through a change in life, which is called "male menopause" or, technically, *andropause*. Resistance and denial of this change is supported by our culture. Inertia and depression are created by the effects of falling testosterone and rising estrogen and contribute to the difficulty. The second challenge is **to take action**. Here is a summary of my recommendations:

1. Reduce abdominal fat and maintain ideal body weight
2. Decrease or eliminate alcohol
3. Detoxify and support liver function
4. Supplement with zinc, at least 60 mg. a day
5. Stay actively engaged in your life
6. Work with a knowledgeable health professional

DHEA

This is considered the mother of all steroid hormones and supplementation can provide many benefits for men and women over forty. These include increased sense of well being, increased immunity, stronger bones and resilience to stress. Women can safely experiment with 10 mg. per day and men with 25mg. A prudent approach is to have all your key hormones tested by an appropriate physician and supplement accordingly. The medical research on DHEA is surprisingly favorable including a good safety record.

Pregnenalone

This is the sister to DHEA and is not only a steroid hormone precursor, but is very helpful for brain function. A safe dose for both men and women is 25 mg. per day. Among its many benefits is that of cognitive enhancement, including supporting memory.

Melatonin

This is the sleep hormone. Its use is controversial but there is good research on its benefits for jet lag, shift work, insomnia, as a brain antioxidant and as a breast cancer preventative. You can experiment with a very small dose, such as ½ mg. approximately 30-60 minutes before bedtime and go up from there. For jet lag a larger dose can be used for a short period of time, up to 1-2 mg. per time zone crossed. Take it before bedtime at your destination. I personally found this very effective a number of years ago on a trip to Europe.

Experimenting Safely With   **Baby Step #28** ☐☐☐
Natural Hormones

Depending on your need, try using one or more of these natural hormones if you are over the age of 40.
1. DHEA – Men start with 25 mg. per day, women take 10 mg. per day. For increased sense of well being, immunity, libido, strong bones and stress reduction.
2. Pregnenalone – Start with 25 mg. a day for men and women, to help with stress, brain function and memory.
3. Melatonin – .5 mg. to 3 mg. daily for sleep before bedtime or up to 1-2 mg. per time zone crossed for jet lag.

Permanent Weight Loss

Many people have been able to lose weight only to gain it right back. Not only is this frustrating and hard on one's self-esteem, but it produces a net loss of muscle mass, making future weight loss that much more difficult. The solution is to confront the source of the problem, which in most cases is an addiction to carbohydrates. If you are among the 64% of the U.S. population who are overweight (or even more importantly, if you are among the 30% who are clinically obese), then ask yourself this question: **"What are my favorite comfort foods?"** In the vast majority of cases these foods are sweets and empty starches, that is, carbohydrates such as chips, cookies, cakes, ice cream, pastries, pasta, breads, etc. *A common but destructive syndrome is to develop an allergy/addiction to your very own comfort foods.* In this case you crave these foods and feel worse when not eating them, and better when you do eat them, even though they may be the cause of many chronic symptoms and health problems (see section on Hidden Food Allergies in this chapter).

After many years of observation and research, I have come to the conclusion that in most cases, successful, permanent weight loss involves radically altering the metabolism to eliminate the craving, dependence and addiction to carbohydrates. The body must be converted from a fat storage machine to a fat burning machine. This is done by eating a specific diet involving low levels of carbohydrate consumption, mainly from vegetables and some fruits combined with "clean" protein and targeted nutritional supplementation. "Clean" protein includes: (1) organic vegetable sources like soy, nuts and seeds; (2) wild fish (non-farmed); and (3) free range antibiotic free chicken or turkey (fowl) and to a lesser extent, red meat.

If you are within 10-15 pounds of your ideal weight, then this may be accomplished on your own through a "zone" type diet (see Baby Step #16) and by moderately increasing your aerobic or cardio exercise. If you need to lose more than 15 pounds, then I recommend working with a professional who has experience with carbohydrate-reduced diets. I have discovered a highly successful version of the Atkins diet called Ultra Lite™. I provide it to my patients and I have found it to be safe and effective, avoiding the pitfalls of Atkins. It is relatively new to this country but is the largest and most successful program of its type in Australia. As far as excess weight is concerned, Australia is the third leading country in the world after the U.S. and England. Ultra Lite has several advantages over other programs offered in this country. It is only provided by health professionals, is reasonably priced and offers a brilliant maintenance plan. To find an Ultra Lite provider near you, call toll free at 1-888-858-7296 or navigate your web browser to www.ultralite.info.

Obviously when it comes to weight loss, there are potentially important emotional issues that need to be addressed as well. Often this can be accomplished through utilizing the Wellness Process™ in Part I of this book. For instance, if weight loss is one of your goals and you suspect you have hidden resistance and are sabotaging yourself (very likely) then pick a Baby Step in question #4 like cutting out junk food and "empty" carbohydrates. Run through the process and see what happens. Pay special attention to all questions in Chapter VI. This will help you break through and control any food addictions and eat in a way that supports your health and ideal body weight. By the way, if you do go off excess carbohydrates cold turkey, then you may experience withdrawal symptoms for the first few days. This can show up as irritability, headache and/or fatigue. Eating a good portion of clean protein at each meal can minimize this (including breakfast) as can increasing green vegetables, especially **Steamed Greens!** This would be an excellent time to review the *Five Key Dietary Principles* in the diet section of this chapter.

Medications

Medications are another good news/bad news story relative to wellness. With some medical conditions, meds can be absolutely necessary for health and life. Some are legitimate medical miracles, like antibiotics and insulin. A dark side exists, however, and here are two examples. First, a major medical crisis is developing because antibiotics have been seriously over prescribed, both for humans and for livestock. Many deadly bacteria have become antibiotic resistant. Second, insulin is life-saving for Type I (juvenile) diabetics but often does little for Type II (adult) diabetics. More and more people are getting the adult form of the disease at earlier and earlier ages, even children. This is a lifestyle disease from immune system insults and too much sugar, refined carbos and lack of exercise. No drug can make up for that.

Some meds are also helpful on an occasional basis or as a convenience, like taking an aspirin for a headache or an antihistamine for hay fever. The scary thing is the dangerous side effects that drugs can have, particularly in the elderly. This is especially true if more than one medication is taken, which is often the case. **Adverse drug reactions with no medical error involved account for over 100,000 deaths a year on a conservative estimate.**[5] If this number is combined with deaths from medical and hospital mishaps, **the total is over 250,000 deaths per year, which makes western medicine the 3rd leading cause of death after heart disease and cancer.**[6] The good news is that medication saves lives and the bad news is that it can take lives unnecessarily as well. As much as possible, rely on wellness, prevention and natural alternative methods to keep you out of the doctor's office and off medications.

Reviewing Your Meds   **Baby Step #29** ☐☐☐

Even if you are taking only one prescription medication on a regular basis, and especially if you are taking multiple meds, then it is critical to review this periodically with your doctor and/or pharmacist! Make a list of each medication and exact dosage you are taking as well as the diagnosis or symptom for which you are taking them. Also include a list of any other symptoms you are experiencing, especially new ones, as these can be **side effects** of your meds. A concise outline of your medical history is always helpful as well. Your life could depend on this!

CHAPTER XI
THE PILLAR OF THE MIND

Instead of frittering away your vibrancy with worry or distraction,
realize your mind and body are inextricably united.
What calms and tones up one, soothes and improves the other.

Marsha Sinetar

Introduction

This pillar is certainly crucial, although all three pillars are co-equal and interdependent. **Experiencing mind and body wholeness is an essential key to wellness.** For convenience, and because of the limitation of language, we include the emotions and spirit in this pillar as well. One's inner or spiritual life is a highly personal affair and it is extremely important to balance and harmonize it with all other aspects of life. *Excellent health requires of us that we "feed our soul" and seek and find a deeper, satisfying meaning to life.*

I am convinced that our values, attitudes and emotions have a profound effect on our body. For proof you don't have to look any further than the medically recognized phenomenon of the placebo effect. It is well known that at least 20-30% of people taking an inert substance (placebo) will find relief and some will even experience side effects. The power of the mind is enormous! Deepak Chopra's book, Quantum Healing, is an inspiring and in depth exploration of this vital topic. Recent research has shown that "merely" focusing the mind and training it in certain ways causes observable changes in brain circuitry that can be physically measured. **There appears to be almost limitless possibilities for healing.** With this in mind, carefully check out the building blocks associated with the mental pillar bellow.

The Power of Affirmations

In a positive affirmation you affirm what is true now, what will be true, or what you want to be true in the future. To be effective it is stated in the present tense, without condition or use of any negatives. It usually starts with "I am " or just "I." A poor example would be, "I will try to eat less sugar so I won't get sick." This contains almost every mistake you could possibly make: (1) you don't "try," you do; (2) you focus on positive steps; (3) you keep your goal in mind, not what you want to avoid; (4) speak in the present tense. How about affirming, "I eat only wholesome foods to create excellent health." The difference in the two examples is obvious.

You can use affirmations for any area of personal growth. It is especially effective when used at the end of the relaxation process (Baby Step #34). **Affirmations can help neutralize core level fears and heal early wounds;** the very wounds you may have uncovered doing the Wellness Process™ that create self-sabotage and maintain your secondary gain. In the past, I had a problem with procrastination, which I discovered was related to a fear of making a mistake. That fear stemmed from a negative love pattern learned from my dad, who was a master procrastinator and also very critical of me at times. To help overcome this tendency, I created the following affirmation: "I take bold and decisive action by trusting my wisdom and my power." I further identified a fear of losing my "nice guy" persona and of being rejected, both big risks for me. So I also affirm, "**I am free** to push buttons, make waves, embrace conflict, appear foolish and be provocative." This affirmation is a little edgy on purpose and breaks some of the rules, but I use it to free up inhibitions and give my "shadow" a chance to be expressed in a safe way.

The shadow is that part of ourselves that we hide, repress or deny. As we are socialized by our parents and later in school, we learn that love and approval are conditional on certain behaviors. The parts of us that are socially unacceptable are stuffed into a metaphorical sack and slung over our shoulder so that we, and no one else, will see them. These parts, or sub-selves, don't go away, but stay hidden, creating self-sabotage and leaking out "sideways" as in Freudian slips and potentially destructive behaviors. See in Chapter VI, the section on Our Human Predicament.

At first I recommend creating a simple affirmation for what you want to become, or want more of in your life. A simple beautiful affirmation to help heal core level unworthiness is, "I deserve to receive love." Say this to yourself silently at different times during the day, both when alone and with others. An especially good time is at the beginning of a hug. As mentioned in the section on Healing Touch, at least three hugs a day is recommended. *You deserve to receive love!*

Creating Affirmation   **Baby Step #30**   □□□

You are free to use any of the affirmations already mentioned or to modify them to suit your needs. There are two main methods for creating your own affirmations from scratch. I highly recommend that you get good at this, as it is a lot of fun and very profitable for your ongoing personal development and good health.

Method 1 – *Going for the Gold.* Here you decide what positive qualities or attainments you want more of in your life, such as health and prosperity. A simple affirmation would be, "I am healthy and prosperous." or, "I attract health and prosperity into my life." or, "I create health and prosperity in my life."

Method 2 – *Reversing a Negative.* This time you listen to and make note of any negative messages or "self talk" you are feeding yourself, like, "That was a stupid thing to say," or, "I don't deserve that." Then rephrase it in the most positive way possible. "I express my intelligence through my speech." or, "I deserve to receive.... " or, "I speak with clarity and wisdom." etc.

In this way, **your affirmations evolve as you do.** As your vision and goals grow, then your affirmations will change to help you become the kind of person that achieves them. See the section on Focus and Surrender, The Art of Conscious Creation at the end of this chapter.

Positive Attitude

"Hey, your attitude is your altitude." Young people say this to express the idea that how "high" you get, how much fun you have, and how successful you become, depends on your attitude. Cultivate an "attitude of gratitude." Remember that who we are and what we have depends upon many other things and people, past and present. Give appreciation to yourself and others and be specific, such as, "I noticed how you took care of that without being asked, that was great." or, "I really appreciate it when you stay focused and get things done."

Once when I was preparing for a speaking engagement, in a calm, meditative state I felt a rush of fear form in my belly that spread up to my chest. It felt like a thunder and lightning storm. This got my attention, and, through self-observation, I retraced the fear back to my strong desire to do a good job and really serve my audience. I was "attached" or identified too closely with achieving a certain outcome or result. In pop psychology lingo, I felt like I was leading with my little boy (inner child) who is very vulnerable and terribly hurt by criticism and rejection. As a matter of fact, I started stuttering fairly severely when I was seven years old. Though I have largely overcome it, speaking in front of people is still a huge challenge. Next, I decided to reframe the situation and visualize leading from the adventurous part of myself, who wants to have fun and excitement and isn't attached to outcome or approval. Instantly I felt my fear subside replaced by calm, confidence and joy. I was able to serve those people well and objectively I spoke fluently without fear holding me back.

This story presents an example of a technique you can use to uplift your attitude and enhance your life. I call it **Reframing**, popularized by neurolinguistic programming (NLP). Whenever you feel an "inappropriate" or "negative" emotion (such as anger, fear, anxiety, embarrassment, irritation, sadness, etc.) and you don't understand why, stop as soon as you can and begin witnessing and observing yourself. Name or identify the feeling and characterize the physical sensations associated with it. Now ask yourself what this is about and try to identify the source. Often this will be one of the "thinking errors" or "mental mistakes" identified by Cognitive Therapy. This system has identified more then 20 such errors that people commonly make. For information about Cognitive Therapy go to one of their websites at www.nacbt.org. For a concise list of these errors or mistakes, go to www.choicesoforegon.com and click on "Choices/Manual" and then on the tab, "Thinking Errors." At this site, the errors have been applied to anti-social behavior but they are applicable to most situations. The final step in **Reframing** is to change your perspective and create a whole new way of looking at or thinking about the situation. For a simple and easy way to gain perspective on a "problem" simply ask yourself this question, "Will any of this matter 100 years from now?"

Reframing   **Baby Step #31**   □□□

I find this technique particularly effective for changing attitudes around emotionally charged situations.

1. As soon as you realize you are having an inappropriate or negative emotional reaction to a situation, stop and become the observer or witness of yourself.
2. Fully experience the physical sensations and characterize or describe them.
3. Trace the situation back in your mind to see if you can identify its source. Often this will be a "thinking error" or an attachment to some particular result or outcome.
4. This is the actual reframe, where you make a new decision or see the situation in a new light. Be creative and have fun with this.

      I want to point out the deep and mysterious way that our attitudes and feelings are connected to our physical health. Dr. Dean Ornish has demonstrated this thoroughly in his book, <u>Love and Survival</u>. Heart disease and cancer patients do much better when they are connected to a loving support system such as a spouse, support group or community. Another attitude associated with increased survival is a "fighting spirit." This is often seen in "bad patients" who are difficult to care for because they are complaining and demanding. Within oneself there must be a strong will and determination to fight the disease and not give up. Of course this has to be balanced with realism and the acceptance of what is happening in the present, whatever the future may bring.

      Next, I want to mention **forgiveness** as an important tool of wellness. Knowing that the past cannot be changed (except in our attitudes towards it) seek to identify people in your past against whom you are holding anger or a grudge. Make every effort to forgive them in your heart of hearts, as the only one being hurt by not letting go is you. This does not mean in any way that you condone or sanction their behavior. Many people who have a hard time forgiving confuse this issue. Forgiving does not mean that you have to like the person or spend time with them. Making choices based on these distinctions <u>IS</u> healthy. **Forgiveness means that you let go of holding onto the anger and**

malice you have toward others as worthless baggage. It is important to realize that they made choices that were beyond your control but on some level made sense for them. **Forgiveness allows you to learn the lessons available to you and to go on with your life.** If your pet dies, you don't keep carrying the body around as it decays and putrefies. You mourn its death in a way that seems right for you and bury and release the body so it can return to the earth. In the same way, forgive those who have hurt or wronged you, learn your lessons, and release the attachment to the pain so it can heal in your body.

The really big step is to forgive yourself for anything from the past, and continuously forgive yourself in the present when needed. Forgiving others in your past prepares you for this crucial step. Forgive yourself for everything and anything. Sometimes in difficult situations it may be necessary to forgive yourself first before you are able to forgive another. Review the circumstances and see what part you played without blame. Now seek to forgive yourself for this and then you may be able to forgive the other person.

It's time to start fresh. The health benefits are enormous. I have had many patients with chronic pain, who for example, did not get better until they forgave their ex-spouse and let go of the anger and hurt!

"If we could read the secret history of those we would like to punish,
we would find in each life a sorrow and a suffering
enough to disarm all our hostility."
Henry Wadsworth Longfellow

Forgiveness   **Baby Step #32** □□□

To get the full healing benefit of forgiveness, make a list of all those from your past for whom you hold anger, resentment or a grudge. Order the list from easiest to hardest to forgive. Start at the top and find a way to forgive what they have done (in your opinion) to hurt or anger you. Completely forgive them in your heart of hearts, say goodbye and release them. If you are having a difficult time releasing those at the bottom of your list, then use the following technique. Write them a letter, for your own eyes only, that you have no intention of sending. First say goodbye to all the hurt and pain. Next, say goodbye to every positive thing about them or your relationship. Finally, and most importantly, say goodbye to any last things you are holding on to about them, about what happened, or anything else that is keeping you "bound" to them. When you are all done you have the option of ritually burning the letter. *Once all others are forgiven from your past, then completely forgive yourself – past, present and future.*

As we because more conscious and aware of ourselves on deeper levels we gain the power to intentionally control our beliefs and attitudes, thus facilitating our own healing.

Meditating Mindfully

Meditation can be approached as a simple and natural technique of wellness. Its written history as a mental and spiritual discipline dates back over 2500 years.

I use the term **mindfulness meditation** here to denote techniques that help one become present in the body and help stop the incessant mind chatter emanating from our ego. This is to distinguish it from reverie, channeling, inner journeying or shamanistic states where the goal may be to leave the body, take flight or explore other inner realms.

There are two main approaches to mindfulness meditation and both have the same end result. **One emphasizes focusing the mind on one thing** like reciting a mantra, following the breath or staring at a focal point (such as a yantra). **The other approach is to be fully aware, just present, without any focus** except consciousness itself. Mindfulness Meditation practice has been called Vipasana, Zazen or just Mindfulness in the Buddhist tradition, and Bare Awareness or the Centering Prayer by some in the Christian tradition. If you don't already have a meditation practice, I recommend that you start by experimenting with both of these approaches, and they can be combined. What follows is a simple, straightforward, integrated approach.

Meditating Mindfully   **Baby Step #33** □□□

The goal is to sit perfectly still with your back straight for at least several minutes a day. You can start by focusing your mind on your breathing, just watching it and letting it come slowly and naturaly. Breathing is a fascinating and unique physical activity where voluntary and involuntary controls overlap completely. So, actually letting go enough to just observe yourself breathing involuntarily can be a formidable challenge. You can also count your breaths, either from one to ten, over and over again, or just count "one" with each exhale. If you have a hard time relaxing or letting go, you can recite the mantra-like affirmation, "I am" on the inhale, and "relaxed" on the exhale. At a certain point during your meditation just stop and observe silently. Be aware of everything going on around you and, most importantly, of consciousness itself, without comment. When you notice that your awareness has wandered off on some "thought train" as I call it, which it most certainly will, then bring your mind back to your chosen focus. Then let go and hold the "quiet emptiness" as long as you can until . . . again, when you notice that you have become distracted by a thought, feeling or image, and the mind chatter starts up again, go back to your point of focus and keep repeating this process without analysis or blame.

It seems obvious that the nature of the mind is to wander around a lot, like a wild monkey. I have been told that even Zen masters have to contend with it. Doing this simple technique regularly has been shown to neutralize the effects of stress, to lower blood pressure, slow the pulse and balance the stress hormones. It can put the ego in its place, balance out the emotions and allow a more authentic self to emerge. I can't recommend it highly enough!

Relaxation and Visualization

Learning how to relax is an essential skill of wellness. Doing breathing exercises and meditation are two excellent tools to help you relax. There is also a popular deep relaxation method that works by letting go of each part of the body in sequence, either from head-to-toe, or toe-to-head. Once a deep state of relaxation has been achieved using the next exercise (or a similar one) then this becomes a great time to practice affirmations, visualization or do other inner work.

I will lead you through a sample process, which you can use as is or later modify and improve for your own personal needs. There are three ways to practice this: (1) record yourself reading this relaxation exercise slowly and play it back when you are ready to relax; (2) have a friend read the relaxation exercise to you slowly in a soothing voice; or (3) look it over and get the gist of it, then lead yourself through it without the book, with eyes closed.

Practicing Relaxation   **Baby Step #34** ☐☐☐

Close your eyes, take three slow deep breaths, and start to let yourself relax (silent pause). Now, as you inhale, say silently to yourself, "I am" and as you exhale say "relaxed." "I am . . . relaxed." (Repeat three to ten times). Become aware of the surface on which you are lying and imagine your body getting heavier and heavier (silent pause). Feel yourself press firmly and conforming into the surface. Feel yourself softening like warm wax or clay (pause). Now start at your toes and let go of them completely. Feel your toes relaxing more and more (pause). Imagine there are corks on the end of your toes that are dropping off, allowing any tension in your body to flow out (pause). Now let your feet completely relax as you get heavier and heavier. Feel the relaxation spread to your ankles and up your legs (pause). Your knees are becoming more and more relaxed as you continue to allow tension to flow out through your toes (pause). Now, deep relaxation is spreading up past your thighs, all the way to your hips and pelvis (pause). Your whole body is feeling more and more comfortable as all your tension is flowing out your toes. Any sounds you might hear from the outside environment only serve to relax you even more. Completely let go of any tension in your buttocks and groin. As you inhale allow your breath to fill your body with good, calm energy, and as you exhale feel any tension flow out with the breath and out your toes (pause). Go deeper and deeper and allow the relaxation to spread up into your low back and into your tummy. Let your belly be soft and open. Let your whole back melt and contour to the surface on which you are lying (pause). Feel the relaxation move up into your chest and shoulders as each breath takes you deeper and deeper. Relaxation flows down each arm into your hands

---

and fingers as you completely let go. Imagine corks on each finger dropping off as all tension flows out through your fingers and toes. Feel your neck letting go as relaxation spreads up into your jaw, face, eyes, forehead, scalp, and the back of your head (pause). Every part of you feels completely comfortable and more and more relaxed. Slowly scan your body for any remaining tension and just imagine it flowing effortlessly out your fingers and toes. Notice how deeply relaxed you are and still awake at the same time. Enjoy knowing that each time you practice this technique it will get easier and easier to achieve this state. (This is a "magical," mellow state for doing inner healing. When you are finished come back as follows.) Count backwards from ten to one and gradually come back to the room. Move your body slightly and slowly open your eyes, knowing that you will feel relaxed and refreshed, ready to continue your day!

With practice, your ability to relax will deepen and you will be able to maintain it throughout your day with great benefit. If you also practice some form of mindfulness these skills will dovetail well and enable you to stay focused and present, to be more joyful and to express more of your creative, authentic self. Eventually you will be able to bring this relaxed mindfulness to all aspects of your life.

Relationships
What is to give light must endure burning.
Victor Frankl

All relationships are best approached with reverence and mindfulness. No other area of life can teach us more about ourselves and where we are stuck. This is especially true of our primary relationship with our spouse or intimate partner. It is said, when the student is ready the guru appears; and if you don't have a guru, then get married. No one shows us our "stuff" like our partner. Rather than defending with blame, denial or passive-aggressiveness, we can look to our own attitudes and behavior and try to improve ourselves. Learn to communicate in a loving but assertive fashion and become a good listener. As Steven Covey says in his book, The Seven Habits of Highly Effective People, "Seek first to understand, then to be understood."

To help prime your communication pump, I would like to offer you two simple but very effective techniques. The first is **Sharing Three Positives Before a Negative,** and the second is **Releasing Withholds**.

Sharing Three Positives   **Baby Step #35** ☐☐☐
Before a Negative

This technique works well if you have been holding onto a piece of negative feedback for your partner and you are afraid you don't know how to say it without triggering them. Set aside some private time, about 15-20 minutes weekly or whatever works for you. You each get a chance to share. **The key is that you must give <u>three</u> sincere pieces of positive feedback before you share the negative <u>one</u>.** The partner receiving the feedback must remain silent and listen in a neutral fashion. This is very important. When both of you have completed your sharing, then and only then can you discuss the feedback, and only if both agree to share. Otherwise, it is recommended that you wait 24 hours, especially if the issue is heavily "charged." An advanced way to finish this process is to share what the "negative" feedback says about you rather than it being about your partner.

Examples: "I appreciate that you were so thoughtful and picked up groceries yesterday after your very busy day." "I am very grateful that you were quiet this morning, and let me sleep in." "I love the way you look at me when we make eye contact." "I was really upset earlier when you left your dirty clothes on our new bedroom carpet."

Advanced Step: "What this says about me is that neatness is very important to me. My shadow here is that when I was growing up I had to share a bedroom with my younger brother who was a slob. I was projecting some anger I still have about that onto you."

Releasing Withholds   **Baby Step #36**   □□□

This technique takes a more direct approach. Here you both take turns sharing withholds, but **the key is that there is no discussion immediately following the process.** The receiving partner just listens with a neutral expression on their face and says, "Thanks for sharing." when the first partner is done. Then you alternate. The other key is that the "negative" feedback or Withhold, is shared with the attitude that it's just "stuff" and you want to release it.   The dialogue would go something like this:

Partner A: "I have a Withhold I would like to let go of."

Partner B: "Would you like to share it?"

Partner A: "Yes. I resent that I had to ask you to change the light bulb three times. I feel like you don't listen to me."

Partner B: "Thanks for sharing that."

Then you can reverse roles and partner B can begin. Now, it is especially important to **not** discuss it for 24 hours so the emotions and tempers can cool off. The next day a fruitful discussion can be held without blame, provocation and escalation of pain and anger, etc.

I would like to share two more essential concepts to healthy relationships that can be difficult and painful at times, but well worth the effort. They will pay priceless dividends if applied. They are **accountability** and **commitment.**

Being Accountable   **Baby Step #37** ☐☐☐

This is about holding oneself or another to their word. This is a marvelous technique of personal growth if both parties in a relationship agree to play by the same rules. The incredible benefit of going through this sometimes painful process is your integrity. Do a regular "check in" process and share when and where you have not kept your word. Offer a simple act of service as a make-up to get back into integrity with yourself and your partner. This is far better than having your partner bring it up or ignore it and sweep it under the rug where it will accumulate and fester.

Committing   **Baby Step #38** ☐☐☐

This can be the glue in any long-term relationship. The power here is that it helps you get past the "honeymoon stage" of your relationship, through the stage of being *at* each other to the joyous stage of being *for* each other. Unfortunately, many relationships do not reach this stage and end in break-up or divorce. Remember, commitments can be re-negotiated, but open communication is essential.

Before ending any long-term relationship think twice, and then think again. Make sure you fully realize that most likely you will just pick up where you left off with your next relationship because you "take your work with you." If you are certain that ending the relationship is the best path then do it consciously and *inflict no pain on your ex on purpose.* Splitting up is difficult enough without blaming and projecting onto the other. Have a clean and clear closure process or several and having a neutral facilitator is ideal. **Remember to work on forgiving both your ex and yourself.**

If you are on the other end of a break-up and feel like the dumpee rather than the dumper, then you have special work to do. Rejection can be extremely painful and can trigger abandonment wounds from childhood. It will usually touch the other, almost universal core wound, of lack of self-worth. See the section called Our Emotional

Predicament in Chapter VI. This is a time to develop your self-love and self-esteem with counseling, coaching, journaling, psychotherapy, etc. There are many resources available including books, support groups and seminars. If your long-term relationship has ended because of an untimely death, then it is especially important to do what is called "grief work." Again, resources are available, though you will have to take the first step and reach out.

Career and Service: Wellness in the Workplace

"This is the true joy in life—that of being used for a purpose
recognized by yourself as a mighty one;
that being a force of nature, instead of a feverish,
selfish little clod of ailments and grievances complaining that
the world will not devote itself to making me happy.
I am of the opinion that my life belongs to the whole community
and as long as I live, it is my privilege to do for it whatever I can.
I want to be thoroughly used up when I die.
For the harder I work, the more I live.

George Bernard Shaw

This area of life is fraught with much difficulty and frustration. Many employees feel they are trapped in an unfulfilling job just to earn a living. One way to approach this is to look at the choices and make a decision. This begins the process of moving from feeling like a victim to feeling like a victor, where you take charge of your own life.

You can leave or you can stay. Either one can be a valid choice, depending on your attitude. You can explore your options of other lines of work, even starting your own business and following your bliss, so to speak. There are many valuable and inspiring books available to help you in this direction. The classic book, which is frequently updated, is What Color Is Your Parachute 2004: A Practical Manual For Job Hunters and Career, by Richard Nelson Bolles. Another great book to boost your "prosperity consciousness" is The One Minute Millionaire, by Mark Victor Hansen and Robert G. Allen. They also have a great website called www.theenlightenedway.com.

You can also accept that your "day job" provides a necessary service in your life – providing money – so do the best job you can. Seek to create value for your employer and the company you work for. It is also important to honor and respect the people with whom you work. You still have approximately 148 hours a week that you are not doing your 40 hour-per-week job. Make the most of that time as well. The question does arise about right livelihood, however. If you are a vegetarian, then working in a meat packing plant is probably not a good idea. If you dislike dealing with money, then perhaps you should not be an accountant, realtor or banker. If you really love being with a lot of people or love being outdoors, then don't get stuck behind a desk in a lonely cubicle. Whatever you do, simultaneously see and increase the service value of it, see how it can help others and own how it serves your personally.

From the point of view of the owner or manager, remember that what is good for the employee is good for the company. The onus is on you to set the tone and create a culture that emphasizes honor, respect and teamwork. Invest in your people and support their health and wellness. This will obviously help your bottom line by saving money through reduced absenteeism, fewer work injuries and lower medical expenses. Expand your wellness perspective to include the environment and our entire society. Create a company that leaves a positive legacy; something that will make your grandkids proud.

The Adventure of Living
Life is a daring adventure or nothing.
Helen Keller

Work as if you did not need the money,
Love as if your heart had never been broken,
Dance as if no one were watching.
An Irish Poet

Live as if you knew you could not make a mistake.
My Future Self, 2023

Two interrelated challenges that I have experienced in my life, and seen in many of my patients, is stress and boredom. They can be viewed as two extremes or polar opposites. They occur when life is experienced passively, when one feels like a victim of circumstance. Paradoxically boredom can be quite destructive and stressful and unrelenting stress (see last section in this chapter, Stress Transformed) can become quiet boring. What's needed is an attitude adjustment or a reframe. I offer you an exceptional exercise that I have personally found to be fun and transformational. It can help you move from feeling like a victum to feeling like a winner or victor.

Victim/Victor Reframing   **Baby Step #39**   ☐☐☐

Have your journal and/or paper handy for this exercise. Think of an event from your past when something "bad" happened to you, where you sustained a loss or injury and where you generally felt helpless, trapped or victimized. Now write it out in a story format. For this first version exaggerate how it all just seemed to happen to you, just a series of circumstances in which you were a **victim**. When done, write down how you feel. To simplify, start with the basic emotions like mad, sad, glad or afraid. Then go on to more complex feelings and judgments like ashamed, depressed, embarrassed, relieved, annoyed, violated, etc. Now for the second part, rewrite the story from a place of choice and personal responsibility. Find a way for you that is basically true, to tell the story where your decisions, actions, non-actions and judgments played a key role in creating the whole drama and its outcome. Here is an example from my own life, first as **victim** then as **victor**.

Example (as **Victim**): When my undergraduate college education ended, some of my friends invited me to travel cross-country in a used van. They built a heavy wooden roof rack to store our luggage on top of the vehicle. Driving along at high speed on the way home, in the middle of nowhere, while I slept in the back of the van, there was a blow out. The vehicle lost control. We rolled several times and came to a stop upside down on top of the roof rack, across the other side of the highway facing the opposite direction. All our stuff was scattered along the highway, the windshield popped out, the doors popped open and we literally rolled out of the van with only minor injuries. We were totally stranded. The whole vacation was ruined and I practically lost my life, not to mention my belongings. The police drove me to the airport and the mother of my friends lent me the money for a ticket home. Telling the story this way, I feel angry and embarrassed, and quite helpless. I also feel afraid that I could have lost my life.

Example (as **Victor**): When I finished my undergraduate college education I decided to join a few of my friends in a cross-country road trip. We bought a used van to save money and my friends built and installed a solid wooden roof rack in which to store our luggage. I neglected to check the tires for safety or to calculate how much weight was on top of the vehicle. I let one of my friends drive on the way home. In between towns, at high speed, I woke up to the sound of a blowout and felt the van roll out of control. I remained calm as the vehicle ended up on the opposite side of the highway, upside down on top of the roof rack. I noticed that some of our stuff was strewn along the highway as the windshield popped out and the doors popped open. We literally rolled out, miraculously uninjured and still alive. Help arrived on the scene and we allowed the police to take us to the airport. I was amazed at how little of my possessions I actually lost and was extremely grateful to be alive. I decided to borrow money from the mother of one of my friends to fly home in style. I created an amazing experience for myself and I learned some important life lessons. This time I feel joy, gratitude and empowerment. I see how my choices created a risky situation, but having survived, I also appreciate the valuable lessons I learned.

Notice that this is not about blaming oneself. Playing the victim has the secondary gain or payoff of avoiding blame and staying in a "safe" but stuck place. In the victor mode it appears that taking responsibility involves receiving blame, making mistakes and failing. Herein lies the key to this reframe. **Taking "responsibility" or acknowledging our "ability to respond" gives us power and facilitates learning life's lessons** so they don't have to be repeated. Let's not play the blame game. **From this active role or perspective of taking control, life is viewed as an adventure and there are no mistakes, blame, or failure.** There are just experiences and lessons to be learned (sometimes about how to not do something.) I find that this attitude relieves much suffering and makes life infinitely more fun!

I know that both boredom and stress will greatly diminish in your life if you actively take on this adventurous attitude. The next exercise involves looking at your present life situation from these two perspectives of victim and victor.

Reclaiming Your Power　　　　　　**Baby Step #40** □□□

Ask yourself, "Is there any part of my life where I currently experience feeling trapped, stuck or victimized?" Proceed as in the previous exercise (the Victor/Victim Reframe) and write two stories. In the first version exaggerate how you are helpless, powerless and/or a victim of circumstance. In the second, take control: explain how your choices or non-choices created the situation and what lessons you are learning. Ask yourself what new choices you could make to get a different result. Remember, insanity has been defined as "doing the same thing over and over and expecting a different result."

If boredom is still an issue for you or you haven't chosen to do the last two exercises, then here is a straightforward technique that can help you break through.

Confronting Boredom　　　　　　**Baby Step #41** □□□

The next time you are feeling bored, stop what you are doing, sit down and just observe yourself. I have noticed the feeling of boredom in myself when I have some free time on my hands and I am not motivated to do anything "valuable." I may even be creating distractions for myself to avoid the boredom, like plopping down in front of the TV or computer and flipping through the channels or clicking through websites. Other common distractions can include eating, shopping, emotional drama and sex. **This is the heart of the matter – being honest and notice when you are distracting yourself to avoid feeling the boredom.** The problem is actually the distraction and the avoiding. By just observing and confronting the boredom, I have found that after a brief period of intensification, the feeling will lift like the morning mist in the bright sun. You may experience some negative thoughts or self-talk involving core wounds like unworthiness and/or abandonment. Journaling may help you get through this but on the other side is self-love and acceptance. Just let go, let yourself fall into the abyss of pain, fear or grief, and you will come out the other side. You will connect with your authentic self, which is the observer and is unfazed by boredom or any other "negative" emotion. From this place you can tap

---

into your natural creative energy and enthusiasm for life. You also can cultivate this part of yourself by practicing Mindfulness Meditation and the Relaxation Process covered previously in this chapter. Trust me, boredom will never be the same again.

Finding Your "Yes" and Saying "No"

This is about finding out what matters most to you. Once you have discovered a deeper "yes" it becomes easier to say "no" when necessary. I have known many people, including myself in the past, who have great difficulty saying "no." This comes up in many types of situations, like over-committing to good causes and other people's projects, donating too much money to charities, impulse shopping and spending time with people you don't really like. It also shows up when people feel like they have to be nice all the time and are afraid of hurting other people's feelings. In the poem called *Initiation* by Oriah Mountain Dreamer, she asks, *"I want to know if you can disappoint another to be true to yourself."* Good question! When you know why you are here and what your purpose or mission in life is, then you will be able to say "no" graciously and you will be respected for your decision. It is valuable to look at the flip side of this. How do you feel around a pleaser or over-committer? Do you lose respect for them and feel uncomfortable or stressed? On the other hand, how do you feel around a person who sets clear personal boundaries and is comfortable saying "no" when appropriate? Do you feel safer and more relaxed? I certainly do.

What lights you up and motivates you to get out of bed in the morning? Beyond all your roles and responsibilities, *where is your passion and why are you here?* Having your life aligned with your passion and your purpose supports your wellness. For most people the key step is spending some time "soul-searching" to find a deeper meaning or inspiration for life. For those of you who tend to over-commit, this is a great antidote. As Steven Covey says, *"It is much easier to say no when there is a deeper yes burning inside."*

At several crucial times in my life, during difficult transitions, I spent some quiet time, usually out in nature, to ask myself these questions. I can honestly say that doing this "work" is what guided me to my career, to finding my wife and "soul-mate" and to writing this book. **To help you with this process I offer you the baby step of identifying your core values.** Another crucial question, "What is your life mission or purpose?" I will leave this for you to ponder and discover for yourself. To help you do this keep this question in front of you as much as possible during your day, first thing in the morning and just before falling asleep at night. In addition, schedule yourself some quiet time, preferably out in nature without distractions, and engage these questions.

Here is a list of values to help you decide which ones are core:

Accomplishment	Focus	Peace
Accuracy	Forward the Action	Performance
Achievement	Free Spirit	Personal Development
Acknowledgment	Freedom to Choose	Personal Growth
Adventure	Freedom	Personal Power
Aesthetics/Beauty	Friendship	Power
Altruism	Full Self-Expression	Powerful
Authenticity	Fun	Privacy
Autonomy	Growth	Productivity
Certainty	Honesty	Recognition
Clarity	Humor	Resilience
Collaboration	Independence	Resolute/Resolve
Commitment	Integrity	Risk Taking
Community	Joy	Romance/Magic
Completion	Lack of Pretense	Security
Comradeship	Leadership	Sensuality
Compassion	Learning	Service/Contribution
Connecting/Bonding	Loyalty	Solitude
Creativity	Mastery	Sovereignty
Danger	Meaning	Spirituality
Directness	Moderation	Success
Elegance	Nature	To Be Known
Emotional Health	Nurturing	Tradition
Empowerment	Openness	Tranquility
Ecology	Orderliness	Trust
Excellence	Participation	Vitality
Excitement	Partnership	Zest

Identifying What Matters Most –   **Baby Step #42** ☐☐☐
Core Values

Look over the list above and check off all the words that seem important to you. Then go back over the ones you have selected and circle the ten that mean the most to you. If you are having trouble deciding, then it may be helpful to time it and force yourself to decide, for example, taking three minutes for each step. Now look over your ten circled values and *pick out the <u>three or four</u> that matter most to you and number them so that they are in order of priority,* with number one being the most important. (Don't worry if you are having trouble deciding because you are free to change your mind at any time in the future.) To finish the process, complete the following statement in order of priority.

My core values are:

(1)_____

(2)_____

(3)_____

(4)_____

If you want to explore this area further and would like to work with a wonderful, professional coach who I personally work with and recommend, then contact Elizabeth Austin, R.N., CPCC through her website at www.insideoutcoach.net. With your core values burning inside you, it becomes much easier to say "no" when appropriate. By the way, I've got this picket fence that needs painting . . .?

Being willing to say "no" allows you to set emotional boundaries for yourself. Personal boundaries are a way to balance the need for emotional safety with the need to stay openhearted and vulnerable. I am sure you have all met someone who has been so hurt emotionally that they are shutdown and unavailable. The other extreme is the person who acts like a doormat, or the "pleaser," always concerned about the feelings and needs of others and not taking care of themselves. If you have a part of yourself like either of these two types, learning when to say **"NO!"** appropriately and when to say **"YES!"** is huge!

Setting Honest Boundaries   **Baby Step #44**   ☐☐☐

Use your journal here and evaluate each day whether you said "yes" when you meant "no" or you said "no" when you meant "yes." Then set an honesty goal and notice your reactions and how people respond. Explore your fears and what the risk of being honest is for you.

The Wisdom of Insecurity and
Other Healing Paradoxes
A false sense of security is the only kind there is.

A poet

They say the only true constant in the universe is change. If that is true then wouldn't it be a good idea to embrace that change? Holding on to the way things were is a major source of emotional pain in our lives. The title of the book by Byron Katie expresses it well, <u>Loving What Is</u>. Of course, what is is a moving target, hence the value of embracing change. One way that we resist change is holding on to a false sense of security. We want and need a reasonable amount of physical and financial security, but I am talking about emotional security vs. vulnerability. The idea that we can insulate ourselves from emotional pain just creates more pain. Actually the opposite may be true, an interesting healing paradox.

I recommend that you not only embrace change but also collect paradoxes and look for the irony in life. To paraphrase my good friend and author, Dr. Rick Kirschner–*at the core of all things, one finds endless irony and paradox. They are the warp and woof, the time and space fabric of the universe.* It could be said that one measure of intelligence is the ability to hold irreconcilable opposites simultaneously. One of my favorite all-time quotes is from Winston Churchill during WW II, describing Russian society, which I apply to all life and the universe. **"It is a riddle wrapped in a mystery inside an enigma."**

It can be extremely rewarding to take emotional risks every day, to stretch ourselves, as it were. This type of stretch involves being radically honest and true to our innermost authentic self. This could be something big, like starting or stopping a primary relationship, to something small, like saying "no" when asked for a favor we really don't want to do.

Emotional Stretching　　　　　　　　**Baby Step #44**　☐☐☐

Pick an area of your life where you feel stuck or realize you are holding onto a certain image or way of being. Set a goal of the number of stretches or risks per day or week you will take, depending on your situation. Keep this up for at least three weeks and record each episode in your journal. Evaluate how you are doing and re-negotiate after three weeks. You can modify the risk or stretch as you grow and get more emotionally flexible or move onto something else. **Example 1:** "At least once per day I will speak up and share what's true for me in a situation where normally I would hold back because of embarrassment or fear of how it will be received." **Example 2:** "At least twice per week I will refrain from buying something on impulse that I don't really need. I will wait at least 24 hours and evaluate it in terms of making do with something else, borrowing or doing without."

Focus and Surrender:
The Art of Conscious Creation

This is all about creating your life the way you want it: health and wellness, prosperity, friendship, travel, a beautiful home, making a difference in the world, etc. The achievement of these goals can be facilitated through the paradoxical union of focusing completely and single-mindedly on one worthy goal at a time while simultaneously letting go of all control and surrendering. This can be summarized in an equation: Focused commitment plus surrendered action equals conscious creation.

Focused Commitment + Surrendered Action =
Conscious Creation

This is a tall order, yet most people can do it. It takes some practice and perseverance. This process of focusing and letting go is analogous to, and can be practiced through, Mindfulness Meditation as presented in this chapter, Baby Step #33.

Recent scientific research has demonstrated that using willpower or "mental force" actually produces measurable changes in brain function and <u>structure</u> (see the book, <u>The Mind and The Brain</u>, by Jeffrey M. Schwartz, M.D. and Sharon Begley). This can best be achieved through repeated effort and determination. Putting all doubt aside is crucial. For me this means trusting that my goal and I are worthy, valuable and will not harm anyone. In effect, trusting that "my is thy will."

After setting a worthy goal, the next step is to take effective action, those "baby steps" in the right direction. It is also useful to ask and answer the following question: *"What kind of person do I need to become in order to successfully accomplish this goal?"* Affirmations can be used here to help you accomplish this. In addition, answer the question in Chapter VI, *"What is the risk or what do I need to face, give up or change to reach this goal?"* As all these pieces come into focus and you become "coherent," then the second half of the equation is applied. Surrender the outcome and once again, trust completely. Another way of saying this is: "Let go and let God." This time trust that all is perfect and whatever happens is the way it's "supposed to be" – "loving what is." **This puts you in the center of the paradox, co-creating reality while surrendering to what is.**

Doing the work as outlined above, takes advantage of an amazing principle of nature. It has been called the **"Butterfly Effect."** It is based on the observation that, in forecasting weather, a slight change in initial conditions can make a huge difference in the outcome. It is said that a butterfly flapping its wings in Mongolia can change the weather in San Francisco. You can utilize this by consciously redirecting or refocusing your thoughts in a direction that supports your goals. This same principle is utilized in what is called **"The Trimtab Factor."** This name comes from the navigational control of huge ocean liners. The rudder controls the direction of motion, but a rudder on a 1000-ton ship is huge and hard to maneuver. So there is this relatively small tab on the rudder that can easily be maneuvered, which in turn, moves the rudder, which controls the ship. **Slight alterations in our daily thinking act as a "trimtab" and can make a huge difference in the direction and outcome of our lives.**

The following Baby Step is a simple technique utilizing these principles and supporting conscious creation. You can easily use it any time during your day. It can effectively be used when you notice that you are "off course" or you are not happy with the way you are feeling, the results you are getting or if you want to redirect your life

Refocusing Technique   **Baby Step #45** ☐☐☐

This technique has three simple steps. The **first step** is acknowledging and loving what is, to actually just be present with what is happening in the moment, honestly and without denial. The **second step** is to briefly focus your mind/emotions on the way you want things to be and how you want to feel. Then make that a conscious choice. In other words, set a new intention on the way you want things to be. The **third step** is to simply let go, observe and effortlessly move in that direction. Firmly setting a new intention or reaffirming a previous one can attract or "allow to happen" what you have chosen.

Example 1: You are having an argument with your spouse and you are not sure how it started, but it seems to be escalating. Step 1: You acknowledge the fight, the hurt and the angry feelings you are experiencing. Step 2: You make a choice that you want harmony and affection to dominate your relationship and focus on that intention momentarily. Step 3: You let go and resume your "interaction" with your spouse. Notice from the witness space if the "argument" de-escalates.

Example 2: You wake up early in the morning and don't feel like getting out of bed to do your stretches. Your bed feels so nice and cozy and there is this warm body next to you .... Step 1: You acknowledge that a part of you wants to stay in bed and how comfortable it feels. Step 2: You reaffirm your decision to get up early enough five days a week to exercise. Today is one of those days. You make a choice, or refocus on your goal or Baby Step, and you briefly imagine how good you will feel once you are up and exercising. Step 3: You let go and notice if you remain in bed or get up and start your morning routine.

This Refocusing technique can be summarized as: (1) acknowledge and witness what is happening, (2) choose or refocus on what you want and (3) let go and observe what happens.

The process of living the life you want through The Art of Conscious Creation:

- ♥ Set worthy goals.
- ♥ Work on yourself to become the kind of person who achieves these goals.
- ♥ Single-mindedly focus on achieving them and take appropriate action.
- ♥ Simultaneously let go of any attachment to the outcome.
- ♥ Use the Refocusing Technique frequently to fine-tune your thoughts and direction.

This process takes advantage of the "butterfly" and "trimtab" effects and, with enough of us doing it, we can create a healthier and more peaceful world!

You are in possession of the greatest gifts in the universe.
You are awake. You are alive. You are free.
Choose wisely and celebrate!

Embracing Death As Ally

To some, the very idea of death and dying is something to be shunned. It is considered one of our taboos, not to be mentioned in polite society and definitely not intentionally contemplated or embraced. Many others have gotten inestimable value from doing just that. If you are among the former group, then I heartily recommend that you look into this issue now.

Throughout this book I have encouraged the practice of mindfulness and conscious choice. Making an ally of death is a crucial step in this direction. Otherwise, death can haunt us from the psychological shadows and energize our fears and inhibitions. When it comes to my subconscious, **I want to stalk my own shadow, not feel like it is stalking me.** I stalk my shadow when I embrace the wisdom of insecurity and live like an "adventurer" or warrior. **This means being willing to follow the truth wherever it leads**, no matter how difficult, even into the face of death, or more likely, ego death. When my shadow gains supremacy, I feel weak and insecure and seek to avoid and deny the truth. Continuing in this vein leads to negative physiological effects and ill health. One of the things that made the master samurai so formidable was their training in embracing death, and hence, their ability to walk fearlessly into battle. At least they were able to conquer their fear and metaphorically place it in front of them on the tip of their sword.

So how does a modern westerner go about doing this important work? I suggest you use the five steps discussed in the previous section on **The Art of Conscious Creation.**

> **Step 1:** Set a goal of making death your ally and consciously choose this.
> **Step 2:** Work on yourself to be the kind of person who achieves this goal, such as courageous, insightful, determined, etc.
> **Step 3:** Single-mindedly focus on achieving this goal and take appropriate action
> **Step 4:** Simultaneously let go of any attachment to the outcome.
> **Step 5:** Use the refocusing technique (Baby Step #45) frequently to stay on track.

So what kind of person successfully embraces death? Look for role models in your life or characters from history, literature or your imagination. Ghandhi, Martin Luther King, Nelson Mandela, Joan of Arc, Yoda and Gandolf come to mind. I would also recommend making a master list of unfinished business and working through the list. This would include the list of people you need to forgive (Baby Step #32) and any other people or things you need to see or do. Ask yourself, "If I were to die tomorrow what would be my regrets?" Said differently, "What do I need to do, say or see such that I will have no regrets on my deathbed?" Letting go of the outcome (**step 4** above), is a helpful skill that can be developed and applied to this issue. It can be practiced daily on small things (like letting go of breath on the exhale during deep breathing), to bigger things like (letting go of ego attachments). A thorough way to deal with death is to set aside a whole year ("god willing") and work through the excellent book by Stephen Levine, <u>A Year To Live</u>. This is especially useful if you go through this with a "buddy" or form a small study group. The book actually includes a month-by-month plan for group practice. I have done this and it made a

my life and greatly diminished my fear of death,
lying. *"Come to your life like a warrior, an'*
(sic)" (from <u>Song Of The Soul</u>, by Cris
**rk of embracing death to empower life and
' journey into wellness.**

---

lly   **Baby Step #46** ☐☐☐

it, look for opportunities to confront the idea of
life as a warrior or adventurer!
and apply the 5 steps of Conscious Creation
section.
ɛd business (including forgiveness) and develop
ɔ.
ɔok, <u>A Year To Live</u>, by Stephen Levine, either
by yourself, with a buddy or in a small group.

Stress Transformed

I have purposely left stress for last. If you have implemented
even one or two of the ideas expressed in this book, then you have
probably already noticed that your ability to deal with stress has
increased. This is beyond mere coping. The concept here is that stress
cannot be completely avoided, although it is beneficial to minimize the
source of it as much as possible. More importantly, we can increase our
resistance or capacity for it through this journey into wellness. In other
words, your stress will appear to go down as your health increases.
There is an inverse relationship between stress and wellness. It is
important to realize that, to reduce the negative effects of stress on your
life, you can work on all three pillars of wellness, not just the mental
one. This means that exercise and nutrition, for instance, also play a
vital role. If you have identified stress as an important health issue, then
take this process to heart and continue to walk with me on this journey
called wellness and don't look back!

Epilogue

A Sustainable Future: Healthy People = Healthy Planet

My hope and prayer is that if you have reached this far, you are well on your way to creating more health and wellness in your life. I believe doing this is necessary, not only for our personal survival, but for the survival of our planet, spaceship earth.

My father warned me back in the early 70's, a long time before the first Earth Day, that I was to beware of the melting of the ice caps, and that someday this would forebode the beginning of the end of our life-friendly environment. I remember hearing, in shock and disbelief, durring the summer of '02, that there was open ocean at the North Pole and that our ice caps were indeed melting. Right now every moment is precious. The fate of the world as we know it hangs in the balance. Act now to create a healthy life for yourself and reach out with forgiveness and compassion to those around you and to the planet itself. The choice is ours–a degrading environment, mass starvation, social chaos and destruction–or a golden age of health, prosperity and the flowering of human creativity with unlimited potential. How each of us lives this day may well decide our future.

> *May be we kind, may we be wise,*
> *may we be powerful and may we be fully awake.*
> *Until we meet again . . .*
> *May the blessings of health be yours.*

Part III

Appendices

APPENDIX A

RECOMMENDED BOOKS AND WEBSITES

What follows is a list of recommended books with my brief comments. They are in the order they appear in the text.

A General Theory Of Love, by Thomas Lewis, M.D., Fari Amini, M.D. and Richard Lannon, M.D.

An amazing book, coming from a heartfelt place, written by three psychiatrists. This book demonstrates the primal and biological importance of love for our health and survival.

Journey Into Love, by Kani Comstock

An easy read, clearly explaining the sources of "negative love" from our childhood wounds. Kani is a Hoffman Process facilitator.

The Art of Sexual Ecstasy, by Margo Anand

An inviting large format book that has been very helpful for many people.

Tantra, The Art Of Conscious Loving, by Charles and Caroline Muir

My wife and I have studied with the Muirs and their book is beautifully written and inspiring.

Mystical Sex, by Louis Meldman, Ph.D.

This book is on my "to read" list and is highly recommended by a "Sacred Sex" teacher of ours, Ulla Angola.

The Chronic Pain Solution, by James N. Dillard, M.D., D.C., C.Ac.

A useful and supportive book compatible with my approach to wellness.

The Zone Diet, by Barry Sears Ph.D.

I find all of Dr. Sears' books useful and full of excellent scientific information about body chemistry. His books provide a solid foundation for a good diet.

The Omega Diet, by Artemis Simopoulos, M.D.
>This is a good description of the Mediterranean diet with emphasis on Omega 3 oils and their many benefits.

Syndrome X: The Complete Nutritional Program To Prevent And Reverse Insulin Resistance, by Burton Berkson and Jack Chalem
>Just what the name says, a very useful book!

The Schwarzbein Principle, by Diana Schwarzbein, M.D.
>This book is very inspiring and has a thorough explanation of how to eat a truly balanced "whole food" diet with good fats and sufficient protein.

The Greatest Experiment Ever Performed On Women, by Barbara Seaman
>Exposes how modern women have been placed at risk because of the greed of the pharmaceutical industry; definitely advocates for women, possibly at the expense of complete objectivity.

The Wisdom Of Menopause, by Christine Northrup, M.D.
>A must-read for both women and their partners. This book thoroughly covers the entire spectrum of body, mind, and spirit issues.

The Mind And The Brain, by Jeffrey M. Schwartz, M.D. and Sharon Begley
>Very exciting research into how our conscious choices or "mental force" makes a real difference in our brain and our life.

Quantum Healing, by Deepak Chopra, M.D.
>A compelling and in-depth exploration of the power of the mind to heal the body.

Love And Survival, by Dean Ornish, M.D.
>A compassionate and scientifically documented explanation of the importance of love and connection in health.

7 Habits Of Highly Successful People, by Steven Covey
>A valuable source of inspiration on living a life based on values and manifesting results in the world.

What Color Is Your Parachute, by Richard Nelson Bolles
The classic book on finding a job or career compatible with your unique talents and sensibilities.

Initiation, by Oriah Mountain Dreamer
This book is based on the wonderful poem by the same author.

Loving What Is, by Byron Katie
Helpful for getting in touch with your authentic self.

One Minute Millionaire, by Mark Victor Hansen and Robert G. Allen
Unique and inspiring both to our rational and emotional brains, placing the generation of wealth in a socially beneficial context.

Life By Design, by Rick Kirschner, N.D.
A fun an exciting approach to creating a healthy, well-balanced life. Highly recommended.

A Year To Live, by Stephen Levine
An invaluable book for helping you embrace death so as to enhance your life. Can be used alone, with a buddy or in a small group.

WEBSITES

These sites are listed in the order they appear in the text with my brief comments. They are followed by other useful links.

www.amtamassage.org -- American Massage Therapy Association
>Very useful and informative, helps in finding a licensed massage therapist in your area.

www.ullalacoaching.com -- Ulla Angola's site
>She can be reached there for more information about sacred sex workshops in your area.

www.amerchiro.org -- American Chiropractic Association
>A great resource: includes summaries of medical research on chiropractic and help in finding a practitioner in your area. I am a member of this association.

www.larreamed.org -- International Larrea Medical Society
>Contains information on the medical research and health benefits of the herb Chaparral (Shegoi).

www.shegoi.net/drkalb -- One of my websites
>Go here to order the special extract of chaparral direct from the manufacturer, Shegoi.

www.metagenics.com -- Metagenics. Inc.
>The largest supplier of nutritional supplements to professionals. Go to this site to find a health professional in your area who provides the UltaClear products and the 4R® gut resoration program. Click on "Contact Us" and send an e-mail to the company with your request for information.

www.ultralie.info -- Site for the Ultra Lite Program
>Locate a health care professional here who provides this reduced carbohydrate weight loss program in your area.

www.left.org -- Life Extension Foundation
>One of my favorite sites for cutting edge and life-saving information about alternative and medical treatments.

www.nacbt.org -- National Association of Cognitive-Behavior Therapists
>A good start for more info about cognitive therapy.

www.choicesoforegon.com -- Choices of Oregon's site
>Contains a useful list of "thinking errors" applied to anti-social behavior.

www.theenlightenedway.com -- Associated with the book, The One Minute Millionaire
>A useful site that supports the generation of wealth in a way that benefits society and the environment.

www.insideoutcoach.net -- The coach, Elizabeth Austin, R.N., CPCC
>Elizabeth is my personal coach. She calls her work "Inside Out Life Design" and she specializes in "Coaching for visionaries and social artists."

www.aapainmanage.org -- American Academy of Pain Management
>This is an interdisciplinary association which is very patient friendly. Locate members here in your locale. Check out their Patient's Bill of Rights.

Additional recommended websites not specifically mentioned in the text:

www.mercola.com -- Dr. Mercola's top health site.
>This is great for keeping up with the latest research on health and nutrition, one of my favorites. You can sign up for his free health newsletter.

www.chopra.com -- Deepok Chopra's website
There are some very nice experiential features, especially "Wisdom Within," a multi-media presentation of body, mind, and spirit information. Dr. Chopra has been very successful in bringing eastern wisdom to the west.

www.drweil.com -- Dr. Andrew Weil's website
Lots of good info and useful tools, many free e-mail updates available. Dr. Weil has brought holistic and alternative medicine to millions.

www.functionalmedicine.org -- Institute for Functional Medicine
A scholarly site where you can search for a doctor versed in diet, detox and the "Four R Program" for digestive health.

www.themeatrix.com -- An extremely clever animation
Shows how factory-raised commercial animal products are produced as a parody of the movie, The Matrix. Don't miss this site!

www.realage.com -- Find out your biological age
Go to this site to take a free test to determine how old you really are. As a whole, this site is a bit too commercial for my liking.

www.ncptsd -- National Center for PTSD.
To find a good article on "thinking errors" click on "Publications," then on "Clinical Quarterly," and scroll down to Volume 7(1), Winter 1997.

www.enhearten.org -- Theohumanity and the ESH Institute
Daniel Baron's work including Emotive Sub-Self Healing is explained here.

Appendix B

Other Resources

MEDICAL SYMPTOMS QUESTIONAIRE

Rate each of the following symptoms based upon your health profile for the past 30 days.

POINT SCALE:

1 = *Occasionally* have it, effect is *not severe*
2 = *Occasionally* have it, effect is *severe*
3 = *Frequently* have it, effect is *not severe*
4 = *Frequently* have it, effect is *severe*

DIGESTIVE	_____	Nausea or vomiting
TRACT	_____	Diarrhea
	_____	Constipation
	_____	Bloated feeling
	_____	Belching, or passing gas
	_____	Heartburn
Total	_____	
EARS	_____	Itchy ears
	_____	Earaches, ear infections
	_____	Drainage from ear
	_____	Ringing in ears, hearing loss
Total	_____	
EMOTIONS	_____	Mood swings
	_____	Anxiety, fear or nervousness
	_____	Anger, irritability
	_____	Depression
Total	_____	

MEDICAL SYMPTOMS QUESTIONAIRE
(Continued)

ENERGY/	_____	Fatigue, sluggishness
ACTIVITY	_____	Apathy, lethargy
	_____	Hyperactivity
	_____	Restlessness
Total	_____	
HEART	_____	Irregular or skipped heartbeat
	_____	Rapid or pounding heartbeat
	_____	Chest pain
Total	_____	
EYES	_____	Watery or itchy eyes
	_____	Swollen, reddened or sticky eyelids
	_____	Bags or dark circles under eyes
	_____	Blurred or tunnel vision (does not include near or farsightedness)
Total	_____	
HEAD	_____	Headaches
	_____	Faintness
	_____	Dizziness
	_____	Insomnia
Total	_____	

MEDICAL SYMPTOMS QUESTIONAIRE
(Continued)

JOINTS/	_____	Pain or aches in joints
MUSCLES	_____	Arthritis
	_____	Stiffness or limitation of movement
	_____	Pain or aches in muscles
	_____	Feeling of weakness or tiredness
Total	_____	
LUNGS	_____	Chest congestion
	_____	Asthma, bronchitis
	_____	Shortness of breath
	_____	Difficulty breathing
Total	_____	
MOUTH/	_____	Chronic coughing
THROAT	_____	Gagging, frequent need to clear throat
	_____	Sore throat, hoarseness, loss of voice
	_____	Swollen or discolored tongue, gums, lips
	_____	Canker sores
Total	_____	
NOSE	_____	Stuffy nose
	_____	Sinus problems
	_____	Hay fever
	_____	Sneezing attacks
	_____	Excessive mucous formation
Total	_____	

MEDICAL SYMPTOMS QUESTIONAIRE
(Continued)

SKIN	_____	Acne
	_____	Hives, rashes or dry skin
	_____	Hair loss
	_____	Flushing or hot flashes
	_____	Excessive sweating
Total	_____	
WEIGHT	_____	Binge eating/drinking
	_____	Craving certain foods
	_____	Excessive weight
	_____	Compulsive eating
	_____	Water retention
	_____	Underweight
Total	_____	
OTHER	_____	Frequent illness
	_____	Frequent or urgent urination
	_____	Genital itch or discharge
Total	_____	

_____	**GRAND TOTAL**

Modified Elimination Diet

This dietary approach has been most helpful with patients who complain of fatigue, recurrent gastrointestinal problems, food intolerance or allergy, chemical or environmental sensitivities, chronic headache, and muscle or joint pain of unknown origin. This diet is dairy and gluten-free and usually well tolerated.

PRIMARY GUIDELINES:

♦ Eliminate all dairy products, including milk, cream, cheese, cottage cheese, yogurt, butter, ice cream and frozen yogurt. Avoid products like soy cheese, which are made with casein (a milk protein).

♦ Eliminate fatty meats like beef, pork, or veal. Chicken, turkey, lean cuts of lamb and cold-water fish (not famed) such as salmon, mackerel and trout are acceptable if you are not allergic to or intolerant of these foods. Select from organic or free-range products whenever possible.

♦ Eliminate gluten. Avoid any foods that contain wheat, spelt, kamut, oat, rye, barley or malt. This is the most difficult part of the diet, but it is also the most important. Unfortunately, gluten is in many common foods including bread, cereal, pasta, crackers and products containing flours made from the above grains. Products made from rice, millet, buckwheat and gluten-free flour or potato, tapioca and arrowroot may be used as desired by most individuals.

♦ Drink at least two quarts of water, preferably filtered, daily.

♦ Avoid all alcohol-containing products, including beer, wine, liquor and over-the-counter products containing alcohol. Avoid all caffeine-containing beverages including coffee, coffee-containing tea and soda pop. Coffee substitutes from gluten-containing grains should be avoided along with decaffeinated coffee. Be sure to read the labels of cold remedies and herbal preparations as they frequently contain caffeine and/or alcohol.

♦ Avoid foods containing yeast or foods that promote yeast overgrowth (processed foods, refined sugars, soy sauce, cheese, commercially prepared condiments, peanuts, vinegar and alcoholic beverages).

Modified Elimination Diet
(Continued)

FOOD GROUP	ALLOWED	AVOID
Meat, Fish, Poultry Legumes Eggs	Chicken, turkey, lean lamb Cold water fish such as salmon, halibut, mackerel, trout, tuna; all legumes, dried peas and lentils	Red meat, cold cuts, sausage, canned meats, frankfurters, eggs, cholesterol-free egg substitutes, egg replacer
Dairy Products	Milk substitutes such as rice milk and nut milk	Milk, cheese, cottage cheese, yogurt, ice cream, non-dairy creamers
Starch	White or sweet potato, rice, tapioca, buckwheat, millet, arrowroot, gluten-free products	All gluten-containing products, including pasta; all corn and corn-containing products
Bread/Cereal	Any made from rice, quinoa, amaranth, buckwheat, teff, millet, potato flour, tapioca, arrowroot or gluten-free flour-based products	All made from wheat, oat, rye, soy, barley or gluten-containing grains
Vegetables	All vegetables, preferably fresh, frozen or freshly juiced	Any vegetables creamed or made with prohibited ingredients
Fruits	Unsweetened fresh, frozen, freshly juiced, or water-packed excluding citrus and strawberries	Fruit drinks, aides, cocktails, citrus, strawberries and dried fruits preserved with sulfites
Soup	Clear vegetable-based broth, homemade vegetarian, chicken or turkey soup; chili made with ground chicken or turkey	Canned or creamed soup, any with glutenous flours or grains
Beverages	Freshly prepared or unsweetened fruit or vegetable juice, pure water, herbal tea	Milk, dairy-based products, coffee, tea, cocoa, Postum, alcoholic beverages, soda pop, sweetened citrus drinks

Modified Elimination Diet
(Continued)

FOOD GROUP	ALLOWED	AVOID
Fats/Oils	Cold, expeller pressed, unrefined, light-shielded-canola, flax, olive, sesame, pumpkin and walnut oil; salad dressing made from allowed ingredients	Margarine, shortening, butter, refined oils, salad dressing and spreads
Nuts/Seeds	Almonds, cashews, sesame, pecans, pumpkin, , flaxseed, squash seeds, sunflower seeds, walnuts, hazelnuts (filberts), nut/seed butters made with allowed ingredients	Peanuts, pistachios, peanut butter, macadamia nuts
Sweeteners	Brown rice syrup, fruit sweeteners	Brown sugar, honey, molasses, maple syrup, corn syrup, fructose, artificial sweeteners
Condiments	Salt-free seasoning and herbs such as bay, caraway, cinnamon, curry, dill, dry mustard, garlic, tarragon, marjoram, nutmeg, ginger, poppy seeds, savory, mint	Salt, soy sauce, mayonnaise, ketchup, etc.

End Notes

[1] JAMA Oct. 9, 2002; 288:1723-1727

[2] Storfield, B. Primary Care: Balancing Health Needs, Services and Technology.
   New York, NY: Oxford University Press; 1998.

[3] http://www.who.int/health-systems.performance/whr200htm

[4] NEJM Jan. 7, 1999; 340:48, 70-76

[5] Kohn L, ed, Corrigan J, ed, Donaldson M., ed. To Err Is Human: Building A Safer Health System.
   Washington, DC: National Academy Press; 1999.

[6] JAMA 2000 Jul. 26; 284 (4):483-5

Dr. Kalb's Bio and Philosophy

Dr. John Kalb and his wife, Shari, have two daughters. They have been members of the Ashland community since 1984. Dr. Kalb holds a Bachelor of Arts degree in Psychology and Chemistry from New York University; a Master of Science degree with emphasis in Developmental Biology from the University of Buffalo and a Doctor of Chiropractic degree from Western States Chiropractic College. He also completed a year of study at the California Acupuncture College in Santa Barbara. He has taken numerous post-graduate seminars in Chiropractic Orthopedics, Clinical Nutrition and other related courses. He actively pursues his continuing education and stays current with scientific and nutritional research. He received his Doctor of Chiropractic degree in 1981 and has been practicing and teaching full time ever since.

The Hippocratic Oath has been passed down through the ages to assure the integrity of medical practitioners. It states, "First Do No Harm!" Dr. Kalb embraces this philosophy. He chose to become a chiropractic physician, following his own research into biochemistry and human physiology. He became convinced that medicine, as practiced today, with its reliance on drugs and surgery, was not consistent with its own Hippocratic Oath. The excessive use of drugs and surgery has many harmful side effects, including death. This is especially disturbing because their use can often be prevented by natural, safe and effective methods. In search of relief for his own health challenges, Dr. Kalb was introduced to chiropractic. Not only did he find excellent health and well being, but he also found his life's calling. Dr. Kalb is proud of being a chiropractor and reminds his patients that Hippocrates himself said, "In illness, first look to the spine." Dr. Kalb's methods of treatment are consistent with the Hippocratic Oath, combining the most safe and effective techniques of chiropractic, osteopathy, physical therapy, exercise, acupressure, nutrition and herbology. **He emphasizes prevention before intervention.** Dr. Kalb believes *the highest and noblest* *calling of all physicians is to educate their patients in the prevention of the health conditions they treat.*

Dr. Kalb is accepting new patients into his practice and he is available by phone for individual consultation and wellness coaching. This includes the Ultra Lite system of weight management, the system of detox and cleansing using the Ultra Clear products and of course his Wellness Process™. He is also available for workshops and public speaking engagements.

He can be reached locally at 541-488-3001and nationally at 888-488-3001. E-mail him at: john@drkalb.com. His main website is: www.drkalb.com.